VISIT LEAN KIDS ONLINE

www.LEANKIDS.com

Enjoy our interactive website along with this book. On this comprehensive online resource we expand on the health information in this book. You will find this website particularly helpful in the following:

- Personalizing your program
- What's new in children's health and nutrition
- New health warnings!
- Forming a LEAN team with others
- Calculating BMI (body mass index)
- Recommended nutritional supplements
- Recommended fitness equipment
- Printing out health and nutrition charts
- Contacting a personal LEAN coach
- Updates to this book

DR. SEARS'
LEAN KIDS

A TOTAL HEALTH PROGRAM FOR CHILDREN AGES 6–12

William Sears, M.D., *and* Peter Sears, M.D., *with* Sean Foy, M.A.

NEW AMERICAN LIBRARY

New American Library
Published by New American Library, a division of
Penguin Group (USA) Inc., 375 Hudson Street,
New York, New York 10014, U.S.A.
Penguin Books Ltd, 80 Strand,
London WC2R 0RL, England
Penguin Books Australia Ltd, 250 Camberwell Road,
Camberwell, Victoria 3124, Australia
Penguin Books Canada Ltd, 10 Alcorn Avenue,
Toronto, Ontario, Canada M4V 3B2
Penguin Books (N.Z.) Ltd, Cnr Rosedale and Airborne Roads,
Albany, Auckland 1310, New Zealand

Penguin Books Ltd, Registered Offices:
80 Strand, London WC2R 0RL, England

First published by New American Library,
a division of Penguin Group (USA) Inc.

First Printing, September 2003
10 9 8 7 6 5 4 3 2

Ⓡ REGISTERED TRADEMARK—MARCA REGISTRADA

LIBRARY OF CONGRESS CATALOGING-IN-PUBLICATION DATA:

Sears, William.
Dr. Sears' L.E.A.N kids : total health program for children ages 6–12 /
William Sears and Peter Sears.
p. cm.
Includes bibliographical references and index.
ISBN 0-451-20976-1
1. Exercise for children.   2. Physical fitness for children.   3. Children—Health and hygiene.
I. Title: Doctor Sears' LEAN kids.   II. Sears, Peter.   III. Title.

RJ133.S43 2003
613.7'042—dc21
2003044554

Set in Adobe Garamond
Designed by Jennifer Ann Daddio

Printed in the United States of America

PUBLISHER'S NOTE

Every effort has been made to ensure that the information contained in this book is complete and accurate. However, neither the publisher nor the authors are engaged in rendering professional advice or services to the individual reader. The ideas, procedures, and suggestions contained in this book are not intended as a substitute for consulting with your physician. All matters regarding your health require medical supervision. Neither the authors nor the publisher shall be liable or responsible for any loss or damage allegedly arising from any information or suggestion in this book.

To our children,
to whom we try to give
the gift of health:

James

Robert

Peter

Hayden

Erin

Matthew

Stephen

Lauren

Joel

Brooke

CONTENTS

PART TWO:
How to Use the LEAN Kids Program

PART III:
Prevention As Part of the Cure

A WORD FROM DR. BILL: MY LEAN STORY

I grew up fat. I remember wearing "huskies," which were the large-size pants fat kids wore in those days. My nickname was "Templeton," from the overeating rat in E. B. White's *Charlotte's Web*. Only because I was also a hyperactive kid did my overeating not lead to extreme obesity. And I didn't grow out of it. Even on my first date with my wife, Martha, I took her to an all-you-can-eat buffet. I figured in case the date was a dud, at least I could eat.

Years later, I paid the adult price for my childhood excesses. On April 22, 1997, I suffered an illness that threatened to shorten my life but instead probably extended it. I underwent surgery for colon cancer, followed by radiation and chemotherapy. As a father of eight, I was motivated, needless to say, to become a survivor.

The question that haunted me at that time was "Why do some people get cancer, a heart attack, diabetes, or other serious illnesses? And why do some fortunate people escape these dreaded diseases?" I imagined that the answers fell into four categories:

- How you live: Lifestyle
- How you move: Exercise
- How you think: Attitude
- How you eat: Nutrition

That's it, the four keys to health and well-being! And those keys created an acronym that perfectly summed up the goal of the program: LEAN. That's how the LEAN Kids Program was born. I loved the term "lean," because it is a power-packed word that means having *just the right amount of body fat for your body type.* Lean is not overfat, nor over-skinny. To be lean means to have strong, fit muscles and to eat in a comfortable, healthy way.

I realized I had discovered a new focus for my pediatric practice. Instead of just prescribing pills for sickness, my goal was to spare other kids from growing up to get adult diseases. I believe a healthful childhood can lay the foundation for a healthful adulthood. I also believe it's easier to change how you eat and live at age eight than at age forty.

First, I needed to figure out how to make my program work. I had to experience it myself. So it was back to the books. Over the next five years I became a student again. "Show me the science" became my motto. Children are too precious to fall prey to the parade of diet and health fads that adults indulge in. I vowed that only scientifically sound advice would go into the LEAN Kids Program.

My home became a laboratory. I personally experimented with lean ways of living, thinking, and eating. Within twelve weeks I noticed a difference, and within six months I was a head-to-toe happier and healthier person. The first changes I noticed were not in my gut, but in my head. I began thinking and seeing more clearly. My brain seemed to be much more focused. My breathing became more efficient. I noticed that my breathing rate was lower, as was my heart rate. Ah, my "Wisdom of the Body" was returning.

Speaking of focusing, one night at a baseball game I realized I had forgotten my glasses, which I always wore to see the outfield scoreboard. I looked up and was surprised to find that I could read the scoreboard clearly for the first time in ten years without my glasses.

Even my nose was working better. I noticed I possessed a keener sense of smell. I could sniff out a smoker at a much greater distance than I could before. One day I was riding in a car through the Midtown Tunnel in New York City. The smell of exhaust fumes began to bother me so much that I was compelled to ask the driver to turn on the air-conditioning system. It didn't bother the other occupants in the car. That's the problem. It should have bothered them! They had lost their Wisdom of the Body. I had regained mine.

I started naturally craving what was good for me and shunning what was bad. It seemed that some little voice inside was prompting me to "do this" and "avoid that." My tastes became more selective as I began to shun junk food and crave healthier fare. Actually, eating became more pleasurable, not less—a perk for old Templeton.

One of the earliest changes I noticed was a "good gut feeling" after a few months of lean eating. After a meal, I felt not hungry, not too full, just satisfied. And when you feel good inside, you tend to feel good all over. Even my joints and muscles seemed to take on new life. Years ago my wife, Martha, had tried to get me to take up dancing. Yet because she was a graceful dancer and I was a klutz, we never could get it together. Since my muscles and joints had taken on new vitality, I took up swing dancing and actually became quite good. We even beat a few younger couples in a swing-dance contest.

I now had the passion to implement the program, and part of this passion was to share what I'd learned with others.

My pediatric practice became my next laboratory. I offered the LEAN Kids Program to interested children, and then I became their coach, working to help them develop new tastes, new thoughts, and new muscles. Over the years I kept a careful journal of what worked and what didn't and, most important, what lasted. What a difference I noticed! I saw fat kids get lean; sad kids get happy; sick kids get well. I saw kids finally taking charge of their bodies and their health. I saw parents and other caregivers taking on the role of lean coaches for their kids. My whole view toward medicine changed—for the better. I became a practitioner of preventive medicine.

In fact, "making a difference" became our family's motto. When our two oldest sons, Dr. Jim and Dr. Bob, joined the Sears Family Pediatric Practice, I gave them a bit of doctorly and fatherly advice: "Your success in life will not be measured by the money you make or the degrees you earn, but rather by the number of people whose lives are made better because of what you did."

Originally, I had decided to write the LEAN Program book for adults. Then I realized that prevention works better than treatment. When children grow up lean, their bodies interpret leanness as normal and they strive to protect these healthy habits for the rest of their lives. While the overweight adult's body fights getting lean, the lean child's body fights getting fat.

Dr. Sears' LEAN Kids is a result of my passion to teach healthy habits to children at an age when their way of living is most open to being shaped—early in middle childhood. I call it a "program" because that's exactly what it does: it programs healthy habits into your child for life.

One day I was daydreaming like a dad and thinking about what legacies I could leave my children. In addition to the usual stuff, I imagined that the last line of my Last Will and Testament might read: *"And to all my children, I leave the gift of health."*

PART ONE

THE LEAN PROGRAM

*What It Is
and Why It's
Important*

1

THE LEAN KIDS PROGRAM
An Introduction

As a pediatrician and father of eight, I've written this book to help combat the three biggest threats to the health of our children between the ages of six and twelve: being overweight, underfitness, and unhappiness. Knowing that obesity has taken over the lives of millions of America's kids, I want to show you how following the LEAN Kids Program can change the way your child feels, looks, and thinks.

Parents, We Have a Problem

Over the past three decades, I've noticed that more and more of my patients are growing up overfat, underfit, and unhappy.

American kids are getting fatter. At no time in history have American children been more overweight. In fact, the Surgeon General recently ranked childhood and adult obesity as one of the primary public health concerns in the United States, second only to smoking. Much of the blame for this rise in obesity lies with the Standard American Diet (which I call "SAD"), which is high in animal fats, unhealthy saturated fats, and hydrogenated oils; low in fiber; high in processed foods; low in complex carbohydrates and plant-based foods; and high in oversugared foods and beverages.

I believe there are several reasons for these alarming trends. Millions of kids today eat many of their meals outside the home. When children do eat at home, it's often processed, packaged stuff and not fresh, whole foods. While watching television, kids are bombarded with advertising that promotes super-sized fast-food portions.

American kids are getting sicker. Among the many health consequences of the SAD diet is type II diabetes (also known as "insulin-resistant diabetes"), which is reaching epidemic proportions in our population and occurring at younger ages. To experience optimal growth, children need diets high in immune boosters, such as the antioxidants in fresh fruits and vegetables and the omega-3 fats in seafood. The SAD diet includes so many sugared beverages and snack foods that it is low in immune boosters and high in immune suppressors.

American kids are getting sadder. Mood disorders, such as anxiety and depression, are occurring in increasing numbers of children and at younger ages. According to a study published in 2000 in the *Journal of the American Medical Association,* the number of children on prescription mood-altering drugs has increased threefold over the past five years. Medication lines at school nurse offices are getting longer as more and more children are taking prescription drugs to either lift them up or calm them down. And increasing studies are implicating the SAD diet in the epidemic of learning and behavioral problems in schoolchildren.

LEAN KIDS SAY

"Mom, can you help me find the TV remote again?
I want to change channels."
—JIMMY, AGE TEN

American kids are becoming sitters. Our children are living in a world that makes it easy to be inactive. From communities with limited parks and recreation centers to increased parental concern about the safety of unsupervised play, barriers to an active lifestyle surround our kids. The reduction in school physical-education classes, an increase in television viewing habits and electronic game playing, and the pace of parents' hectic schedules all contribute to our children's situation, sitting more and moving less.

Scary Fat Stats

- Between 15 percent and 25 percent (depending on ethnicity) of American children are overfat—triple the rate of thirty years ago.
- For each of the last three decades (1970–2000), the number of overfat children has increased by more than 40 percent from the previous decade.
- Children aren't necessarily eating more fat, but they are eating more unhealthy fats, such as saturated and hydrogenated fats.
- The average child consumes more than 12 ounces of sugar a day, which represents a tremendous increase of daily sugar consumption from twenty years ago.
- While packaged foods are becoming lower in fats, they're becoming higher in sugars.
- Children who are overweight at six have a 25 percent chance of becoming overweight adults. If a child remains fat until he is twelve, the chance of becoming a fat adult increases to 75 percent. Eighty percent of obese adolescents remain obese as adults.
- More people die each year from obesity-related diseases than in war and accidents.
- In the past two decades, obesity rates have doubled, portion sizes have doubled, and the percentage of each food dollar spent and the amount of food eaten outside of the home have doubled.
- From 1979 to 1999, in children ages six to seventeen, hospitalizations for obesity-related diabetes doubled, gallbladder disease tripled, and obesity-related sleep apnea increased fivefold.
- A 1999 study reported that 60 percent of overweight five-to-ten-year-old children already had at least one risk factor for cardiovascular disease, such as high blood pressure, elevated insulin levels, or high blood lipids.

- Children are drinking 23 percent more soft drinks than they did in the late 1970s. Studies show that the more sweetened beverages a child drinks, the more overweight that child is likely to be.
- In the past few decades, fast-food portions have doubled in size. In 1957 a bottle of soda was eight ounces. Nowadays it's a whopping 32 to 64 ounces.
- For the first time in history, obesity has been officially classified as a disease by the American Medical Association, and it now has its own insurance code.
- If the current trend continues, obesity researchers predict that by 2008 *40 percent* of adults will be obese (meaning thirty or more pounds over a healthy weight).

Parents, we have a problem. If these trends continue, America's children face a future filled with sickness rather than health, of weakness rather than strength, of sadness rather than happiness. I'm concerned that if this unhealthy and unhappy trend continues, kids will have a shorter life expectancy than their parents do. What is even more tragic is that the "health expectancy"—the number of years lived in good health—is likely to be less for today's kids.

Parents, We Have a Solution

What we need is a total health program to stop and reverse these alarming trends, just as we have programs to vaccinate younger children against diseases and to teach teens about sex. The LEAN Kids Program is a result of my passion to teach healthy habits to kids, ages six to twelve, when their way of living is most open to being shaped—early in middle childhood. I call it a "program" because that's exactly what it does: It programs healthy habits into your child for life.

Being lean means having just the right amount of body fat for your body type. Becoming lean involves not only trimming unneeded and unhealthy fat from a child's body, but also aims at breaking unhealthy lifestyle habits that interfere with the mental and physical health of your child. I'll show you in the LEAN Kids Program how moving around more (even walking the dog in the neighborhood) can help your child be lean and fit.

The LEAN Kids Program promises to guide your child down the path of health. It is a comprehensive plan that helps children reach their optimal health in twelve weeks. The plan addresses the child's Lifestyle, Exercise, Attitude, and Nutrition. As you read through the program, you will see that it quickly moves from an explanation in Part One of how the program works to page after page of practical advice for living the LEAN Kids Program in Part Two.

Each of the major chapters in Part Two will explain how the LEAN Kids Program works in the four key areas of your child's life.

Lifestyle—Live Lean. This section of the book addresses how your family lives. The goal of the lifestyle part of the program is to empower

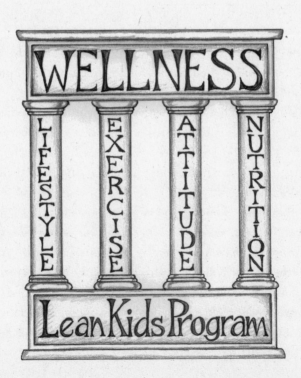

your child to make healthy choices and learn healthy habits. You will learn tools to help you be your child's lean coach and teach your child to take personal responsibility for her health.

Exercise—Play Lean. This section shows you how to get your child moving, not only with regular play activities and family recreation, but also by adding a sport to your child's life and exercise routines to your home. You will learn how to make fitness fun for the entire family.

Attitude—Think Lean. This section will help your child develop a positive attitude about health. You will learn how to help your child understand and like his or her body; to stop negative thinking and enjoy positive thinking; to relax and manage stressful situations.

Nutrition—Eat Lean. This section will empower a child to make wise food and eating choices that enhance his health and well-being. It will show you and your child what and how to eat for optimal health.

What the LEAN Program Is Not!

The LEAN Kids Program is *not* a deprivation weight-loss diet. It's not healthful for children to *lose* weight. Rather, most overfat children should lean out by maintaining their weight for a period of time, until they grow into their body size.

The LEAN Kids Program is *not* a strict menu plan, because children don't eat that way. It is *not* a calorie-counting diet, because it is not realistic to believe that children in this age group will accurately count calories, nor even report accurate enough information about their eating for parents to do it for them.

Besides (and this is one of the most important things I want you to learn from this book), *children don't get fat from eating too much; they get fat from eating too much of the wrong foods and not being active enough.* That's why the LEAN Kids Program redirects the child's cravings toward healthy eating and living habits. Because it is not a restrictive eating plan, it won't damage your child's emotional or psychological relationship with food. It is not the kind of restrictive menu plan that can lead to intense cravings and eating disorders. Rather, it is a balanced program that helps kids start to enjoy and appreciate food more.

That's one reason the LEAN Kids Program is also appropriate for underweight children. While they are not the focus of this book, the truth is that you can help your children increase their weight to a healthy level by following the LEAN plan.

On a more personal note, I am particularly sensitive to the importance of identifying high-risk kids and taking lean action early—because I didn't! When one of our children was at the 85th percentile for weight yet only at the 50th for height at her five-year checkup, Martha asked our pediatrician, "Should I be worried about her weight?" The pediatrician took Martha aside and admonished her not to do anything about the situation. "If you obsess about her weight, you'll set her up for an eating disorder," she advised.

Until recently, that was the party line among pediatricians. We were so afraid of causing eating disorders that we overlooked the fact that more children suffer dire medical consequences from obesity than have nutritional deficiencies from eating too little. While both concerns are important, our view of them has to remain balanced and the individual child has to be taken into account. In chapter 5, I'll show you in detail how to evaluate your child's weight and health, how to personalize the program, and how to choose the course of action appropriate for your own child's state of health.

Here's to Your Child's Health

Is your child overfat, underfit, or unhappy? Does he dread participating in active sports because of his weight and a fear of being teased? Is she moody and unhappy because of being overfat, and does she turn to high-fat junk foods for comfort? It doesn't have to be this way!

In more than three decades of treating children, I have learned a lot about what keeps kids fit and healthy. Now, through the LEAN Kids Program, I want to help parents recognize the early signs of their kids' becoming overfat and underfit, and to teach them how to be proactive with their children in preventing these problems and the unhappiness and ill health they lead to. I want parents to see how improving the lifestyle and diet of their children will improve the health, fitness, and mood of the entire family. Above all, I want parents to keep America's children from becoming unhealthy adults.

Parents, when your children are between the ages of six and twelve, you have a special window of opportunity to teach and model healthy living and eating lessons for them. This age is often described as the last stage in a child's life that he will really listen to his parents' advice. Children under six may not be able to comprehend the full importance of health and nutritional principles. Children over twelve may be unwilling to listen.

Start today. Take advantage of this impressionable time to give your children a successful road map to lean living and optimal health. The LEAN Kids Program shows you how.

Let's get started!

2

GROWING UP LEAN

The Difference

The first step in starting to live a lean life and raising lean children is to learn why it's so important. In the following chapters, we'll discuss this in great detail. Yet I want to first give you a general overview of the importance of lean living.

Suppose you could give your children a pill that could help them be healthier, smarter, happier—that would make them run faster, miss less school, be nicer, live longer, and grow to avoid diseases like diabetes, heart disease, stroke, arthritis, and cancer.

Sound like a fantasy? Well, there's no such pill. But you *can* give your children these gifts. They are the benefits of lean living, and the LEAN Kids Program will show you how to make them part of your life. Lean medicine doesn't come in pill form. Rather, it's made up of many individual *lean choices,* which you can think of as small, frequent doses of medicine that you can give your children throughout each day. At first you'll have to guide your children toward this "medicine" by making a lean choice. But after a while your children will learn to take this "medicine" on their own. Then you can sit back and watch your children enjoy one of the most precious gifts you can give them—the gift of health.

That's what the LEAN Kids Program is all about.

Are You Giving Your Child the Gift of Health?

As parents, we all hope to give our children the tools to succeed in life. But what exactly does that mean?

One day I was discussing this very question with a group of parents. We were specifically talking about what parents can do to help their children succeed in life. Some parents suggested that self-discipline and a good education were most important. An investment banker naturally mentioned money, believing that a savings plan for college was important. Another parent felt that politeness, empathy, and kindness were most important.

When it was my turn, I said, "I think one of the most important things you can do for your children is give them the gift of health." I went on to explain that a healthy child is a privileged child who grows up with an emotional, physical, social, and intellectual advantage.

The other parents looked surprised. They had never thought of health as a gift they could choose to bestow on their children. Then one mother asked, "What do you mean by giving them the gift of health? Do you mean we should keep their immunizations up to date?"

"Immunizing your child against tetanus, polio, diphtheria, measles, and other diseases is important," I replied. "But that's not the only thing you can do for your children. Let's take a walk through your kitchen and I'll show you how you can immunize your children against the diseases of the twenty-first century, such as anxiety, depression, diabetes, cardiovascular disease, arthritis, and some cancers."

Again, the parents were surprised. They had never imagined they could protect their children against these dreaded diseases. They all wanted to know what the "vaccine" against these diseases was. My answer: The LEAN Kids Program.

WHAT LEAN MEANS

Lean means having the right percentage of body fat for your individual body type. Neither too much nor too little body fat is healthy. Lean does not mean thin or skinny, which is often not healthy, since a skinny or underweight child may sometimes be undernourished. For some kids, lean can mean being pretty big.

As I'll discuss more in chapter 5, some children are born big and some are born petite. Size itself is not really the issue. What's more important is that we all have the appropriate amount of muscle for our skeletal frame. Lean means being strong and healthy.

The younger a lean child is, the easier it is to stay lean. Studies show that the older the obese child is, the more likely that child is to become an obese adult. Why would that be the case? If a child lugs around a lot of excess fat during most of his childhood, his body will grow to interpret this excess fat as normal. And the body fights to protect what it considers normal, which is why so many adults struggle and fail in their efforts to lose weight. Prevention is the most effective treatment of obesity.

The child who grows up lean has the advantage of the body interpreting leanness as normal and weight gain as abnormal. In a sense, his or her body becomes internally programmed to protect leanness. This internal programming is called the "Wisdom of the Body."

LEAN KIDS SAY

"I waddle when I walk and my tummy jiggles
like a bowl of Jell-O. I hate that."
—AARON, AGE NINE

THE WISDOM OF THE BODY

Harvard physiologist Dr. Walter Cannon formulated this biochemical principle in 1932. According to the Wisdom of the Body principle, the body is biochemically programmed to eat and do what is good for it and to shun foods and activities that are bad for it. The body believes that the foods that you grow, hunt, milk, or fish are healthy foods, and any other edible substances are unhealthy foods. The wise body, therefore, naturally rebels against processed foods and chemical additives.

I like to think of the Wisdom of the Body as our natural inner *sensitivity,* or a sort of radar system that keeps the bad stuff out. Sadly, many of us have lost touch with this naturally protective shield. But most mothers know what I'm talking about when I discuss the Wisdom of the Body, because pregnancy is a time when many women regain it. An expectant mother becomes exquisitely sensitive to what's good for her own body—and the growing body inside—and will take drastic measures to protect her precious preborn baby.

The LEAN Kids Program is another way you can regain your natural Wisdom of the Body. It will help you and your children become more sensitive to what you eat and the lifestyle choices you make, and it will come to protect you just as a pregnant mother protects her unborn child.

A Tale of Two Kids: Fat Freddy and Lean Lucy

To help give my patients a better sense of what's involved in lean living, I often tell a story about two children, one I call Fat Freddy and the other I've named Lean Lucy. I've made these two kids up to illustrate and summarize some of the most important lessons of the LEAN Kids Program.

Freddie grew up fat. Even when he was a baby, his parents would encourage him to finish the bottle. They treated every whimper as a cry of hunger, and into Freddie's eager mouth a bottle quickly went. At four months, Freddie graduated from formula to his first foods—packaged baby food. So Freddie's first tastes of food during the impressionable first year of life were foods in cans and boxes.

Lucy grew up lean. She was breast-fed when she was hungry and stopped when she was satisfied. At six months, Lucy was given baby food that her mother made from scratch. Sometimes when Lucy fussed, she was held and played with. Sometimes that cheered her up before she was even offered food, so she didn't grow up eating as a response to every discomfort.

Lean Lesson: Shape young tastes early.

As a toddler, Freddie grew fatter. Following his first course of artificial baby foods, Freddie continued his steady diet of packaged foods. His parents believed it was good discipline to get him on a schedule of three big meals a day. Because Freddie became a picky eater, his frustrated parents began the "just one more bite" pleading. They felt desperate for Freddie to clean his plate so he wouldn't be skinny.

Lucy stayed lean. Between the ages of one and two, Lucy lost some of that extra first-year baby fat and began the natural stage of leaning out. Lucy's parents believed their job was to choose nutritious foods and prepare them creatively. When and how much food Lucy ate was up to her.

Lean Lesson: Children (not their parents) should control when and how much they eat.

Freddie grew fatter. When he was a preschooler, his parents continued to push three big meals a day. He was continually served big helpings on adult-sized plates and encouraged to finish them, especially since he continued to be perceived as a picky eater. He ended up always feeling either too hungry or too full. Freddie never felt just right.

Lucy grew lean. Lucy's parents knew tiny children have tiny tummies, about the size of their fists. Early on, the three-big-meals-a-day pattern was scrapped and Lucy was allowed to nibble on *nutritious* foods throughout the day, in addition to enjoying the scheduled meals at the family table. Her parents would put small dollops of food on a small plate and refill as Lucy cued them. Lucy was seldom hungry and rarely felt stuffed. She just felt satisfied after she ate.

Lean Lesson: Raise a grazer.

Freddie went to a fat school. When he entered the school cafeteria, he felt right at home. Cupcakes competed with salads for Freddie's lunch money. Fat-soaked French fries were Freddie's veggie. School vending machines served the same sweetened drinks and soda he gulped at home. His eating habits at home were reinforced by the ones he learned at school. Freddie's family ate out a lot, so his tastes were shaped by his family's four main food groups: McDonald's, Burger King, Pizza Hut, and Kentucky Fried Chicken.

Lucy went to a lean school that focused not only on SAT scores but also on FAT scores. Her parents joined the PTA and successfully lobbied for salad bars and other healthy fare in the cafeteria, and got the soda and junk juice out of the school vending machines. At school, Lucy recognized the healthful foods she ate at home. Lucy's family went out only on special occasions, figuring they could make more healthful choices at home than at a food-for-profit local fast-food outlet.

Lean Lesson: Lobby for lean schools.

When Freddie ate dinner at the homes of lean families, he didn't like the food. He shunned fish. (Packaged goldfish crackers were the only "fish" he had tried.) He rarely ate anything green. But if he had dinner at another "fat home," he felt comfortable with the processed foods and sugary beverages that were served.

When Lucy had dinner at the homes of lean families, she always enjoyed the meal. Lean food had become her norm. To her shaped tastes, the fresh vegetables and the lean fish and meats that the lean families served were simply what normal food was supposed to taste like. Yet when she ate at fat homes, she didn't like the food. She would complain that it made her tummy feel "yucky." Even by the age of eight, Lucy had made the physiological connection, "If I eat well, I feel well."

Lean Lesson: Form a lean team of friends.

Freddie's mom was a "fat shopper." His family frequented the center aisles of the supermarket, where all the packaged goods are displayed. Freddie chose cereal based on the cute pictures on the front of the box. His mom never checked the label for sugar content or other nutritional information.

Lucy's mom was a "lean shopper." She shopped the perimeter of the store, which displayed lean food, such as fresh produce, fish, eggs, lean meat, and dairy products. When Lucy wandered down the packaged-food aisles and chose a cereal, her mother took the opportunity to teach her a food lesson. She advised Lucy not to trust the front of the box, but rather to look at the ingredient label on the side or back of the box. She showed Lucy how to look for words like "whole grain" to be listed first among the ingredients. She told her to avoid foods that listed sugar as the first ingredient, because that told her the food would be mostly made of sugar. She also told Lucy to watch out for words like "hydrogenated" and "red #40," which meant the food had stuff in it that could make her sick.

Lean Lesson: Shop the perimeter of the supermarket.

Freddie's family sat a lot. Freddie sat a lot, too. Mindlessly munching while watching TV was a regular family activity, and Freddie ate when he got bored. The family (and Freddie) grew fatter. He felt different. (To a child, feeling different equates with feeling bad.) He ran slower and tired faster than other eight-year-olds on the soccer team. Because he wasn't good at sports, he hated playing them. Freddie quit the team and became a spectator, or sat by a tree playing his Game Boy while the other children ran. Not only did Freddie look fat, he felt fat. It wasn't fun to run— it was work. So he sat and stayed fat.

Lucy's family moved a lot. They took family walks and played yard games. Except for munching on nutritious snacks while watching TV, mother maintained the rule, "We only eat at the dining table." Father had a "moving equals sitting" rule, which meant that Lucy could watch TV or sit in front of a computer screen only for a time period that matched the same number of minutes she spent actively playing. The family stayed lean. Lucy loved to run. Because it felt good, she ran more and stayed lean.

Lean Lesson: Get kids moving!

Freddie began the day by eating dumb. He skipped breakfast, or at best managed to gulp down a glass of junk juice and a sugary pastry. An hour later, his brain ran out of fuel, so he couldn't sit still and pay attention. By lunchtime Fat Freddie was famished, so he overcompensated for his missed morning meal by pigging out at lunch.

Lean Lucy began the day by eating smart. Breakfast was the most balanced meal of her day, packed with protein, fiber-filled carbs, and just the right amount of healthy fats. Her brain remained charged up all morning and, with the help of a midmorning apple, she felt comfortably hungry at lunchtime.

Lean Lesson: Serve your child a brainy breakfast.

Freddie ate too fast. Because he wolfed down his meals, he didn't realize soon enough when he had eaten enough, and he kept right on eating—too much.

Lucy ate slowly. Her mother reminded her to chew her food thoroughly. And the family talked between bites. Once full, her stomach had time to get the message to her brain that she was satisfied, and she stopped eating—before she ate too much.

Lean Lesson: Eat mindfully.

Freddie loved fat drinks. If it wasn't full of sugary syrup and served in a big container, Freddie wouldn't drink it. His favorite was the supersized soda pop at the neighborhood junk-food store.

Lucy loved lean drinks. Water was the family drink, occasionally flavored with 100 percent juice. When Lucy asked her mother if she could have a big bottle of Junk-O Juice, her lean mom responded, "We don't drink that stuff in our house. It's just chemically colored sugar water, and it will make you feel yucky." One day at a friend's house, Lucy was served a carbonated soda. She took a few sips and thought it tasted odd. She couldn't drink it. Lucy's body was programmed to make the connection "When I eat yucky, I feel yucky."

Lean Lesson: Water your growing child.

Freddie grew up sick. He tired easily and often missed school. By the time he was eleven, his parents felt that he needed a thorough medical evaluation. After the exam and a battery of tests, his pediatrician described to his parents Freddie's problems system by system. "No, it's not his thyroid. Freddie just sits too much and eats too much of the wrong foods. It's as simple as that. He gets sick and misses school often because obesity depresses immunity. He falls asleep at his desk because being obese interferes with normal breathing during sleep, keeping him from enjoying a restful night. His feet and hips hurt when he runs because his growing bones are fatigued from lugging around all that extra weight. And, I'm sorry to say, Freddie is on the verge of getting diabetes."

"Diabetes!" The parents were shocked at hearing the D-word. "But we thought diabetes made you thirsty, skinny, and really sick. Freddie has none of these symptoms."

Their doctor went on to explain, "He doesn't have the type of diabetes you are familiar with, at least not yet. He doesn't need insulin shots. What is happening in Freddie's body is that too much excess body fat is keeping insulin from doing its job. He is insulin resistant and has what is described as type II diabetes, or what used to be called 'prediabetes.' Eventually, Freddie's overweight will overwork his pancreas, and it's likely to wear out from being overfat and underfit all these years. Then he's likely to develop type I, or insulin-dependent, diabetes."

Freddie became an adult. Despite trying various diets, at forty Freddie was still fat. During critical periods in his childhood growth, lifelong unhealthy eating habits had been so imprinted upon him that they were hard to break, and even harder to replace with healthier habits. Freddie's body was so used to being fat that it perceived the excess weight as normal for him. Consequently, his body fought harder to keep the fat on than Freddie could fight to take it off.

Because Freddie was smart, he had managed to compensate for his portly appearance by landing a high-paying job. In fact, he had fed so many assets into his portfolio that he planned to retire at fifty. However, between forty and fifty years of age, Freddie's body began to fall apart. Instead of the good life Freddie had saved for, his social calendar was cluttered with one doctor's appointment after another. Full-blown diabetes set in, which left him tired, grumpy, and wearing thicker and thicker glasses to compensate for his deteriorating vision. Not only did Freddie have vision problems, but he also had difficulty walking because of arthritis. At fifty, Freddie joined the growing numbers of fat executives and had a life-saving triple-bypass surgery for his fat-weakened heart. Like many fat people, he had a chest scar that was like a brand from living an unhealthy childhood.

Freddie didn't live long enough to enjoy his retirement or his grand-children, or even to walk his daughter down the aisle as father of the bride. If he had begun living lean at five, he probably would have lived— and lived well—way beyond fifty.

Lucy grew up well. She seldom got sick, and when she did get sick she recovered quickly. Her brain was focused at school, and she grew up enjoying sports. She grew up to be a lean teenager and a lean adult. Her body was programmed for leanness as her norm, so much so that it rebounded from the occasional lapse in lean living. There seemed to be a little voice inside of Lucy prompting her to make lean choices. Simply put, she felt good when she lived and ate lean, and felt bad when she didn't. Unlike those of her less lean friends, her pregnancies were not complicated by gestational diabetes, and as she aged, Lucy bypassed the obesity-related diseases of heart disease, stroke, and diabetes.

Lucy had a healthier retirement plan. Because she didn't suffer from obesity-related arthritis, she continued to enjoy playing tennis and taking walks. Lucy continued to live the lean life and passed on a legacy of lean living to her grandchildren. Because Lucy lived lean, she lived longer— and healthier.

Lean Lesson: Lean equals longevity.

Few families have as many bad habits as Fat Freddie's, and even fewer are as consistently perfect as Lucy's. We all fall into a spectrum of good to bad family health habits. The sad news is, with 60 percent of Americans overweight, more of us are living like Fat Freddie than like Lean Lucy. And it's time for you to figure out just where your family is in this health spectrum.

As you read on, you will gain greater insight into how kids today get overfat, underfit, and unhappy. In my experience, once parents recognize the cause of the problem, they can use the tools in the LEAN Kids Program to ensure leanness throughout their child's lifetime.

LEAN TIP: KIDS ARE RESILIENT

"But what if I haven't given my child all these lean tips and have unknowingly raised a Fat Freddie?" you may wonder. Don't worry. Kids are resilient. *It's never too late to start.* In all aspects of child development, even going from fatness to leanness, children can overcome a shaky start and go on to lead a leaner and longer life. But the earlier you start, the easier it will be for the whole family to get lean.

3

HOW KIDS GET OVERFAT, UNDERFIT, AND UNHAPPY

The Causes

Now that you have an overview of what I mean by lean living and why it's important, you know how crucial it is to raising happy and healthy children. But the first question parents usually have is, When did this problem get to be so bad? Children weren't always overfat, underfit, and unhappy in epidemic numbers. What's causing these problems to become so serious now?

So let's take a minute in this chapter to talk about the causes of the problems threatening our children.

How Kids Get Overfat

In most cases, kids don't get overfat because they eat too much. They usually get overfat because they eat the wrong foods and don't move enough. It's as simple as that. But what's causing kids to eat so much of the wrong foods and to move so little? Well, the world has changed. And many of the changes that are part of our modern lifestyle have not been good for our health.

For instance, once upon a time kids ran for entertainment—playing catch, ball games, and capture the flag. Nowadays, they *sit* for entertainment—playing Game Boy and X-Box and watching TV. Once upon a time kids ate most of their meals in Mom's kitchen, and Mom's motives in preparing meals were simple—serve whole foods for the better health of her children. Nowadays "kids' meals" are something we get in fast-food outlets, and most franchises are motivated by profit to serve the cheapest food at the lowest cost. Even if we eat at home, today's parents are overscheduled and often turn to time-saving, factory-packaged foods that are usually high in calories, yet low in nutrition.

The truth is that our culture's new dependence on easy-to-prepare fast foods is just one of the reasons our kids are overfat and underfit. But I think it's the number-one reason, so let's start by taking a closer look at packaged foods.

FAT CORPORATIONS

I believe obesity is mainly a shopping problem. *If you buy it, kids will eat it.* So if you're going to buy packaged foods, you should know what goes into those brightly colored boxes. To find out, let's make an imaginary visit to the boardroom of a packaged-food company where they are planning to launch a product for your kids.

Welcome to a board meeting at Junk Food, Inc. The CEO, Mr. Junko, calls the meeting to order by announcing the introduction of a new snack food, appropriately called Junkos.

"Miss Stats," the CEO asks, "what does your market research tell us about kids' eating habits?"

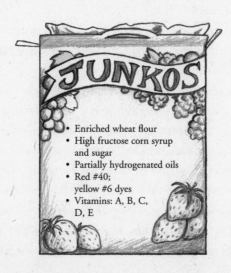

JUNKOS

- Enriched wheat flour
- High fructose corn syrup and sugar
- Partially hydrogenated oils
- Red #40; yellow #6 dyes
- Vitamins: A, B, C, D, E

"Parents don't have time to cook," Miss Stats reports. "Families eat on the run. And when kids aren't racing off to school or to an after-school activity, they sit a lot, watching TV or some computer screen as they mindlessly munch."

Mr. Junko asks, "How can we use these trends to fatten our profits?"

Mr. Sales comments, "Let's bypass parents and pitch our products directly to kids. Lots of parents are getting health-conscious nowadays, so that's not our market. Let's advertise on the kids' TV programs. We'll show kids gorging themselves with handfuls of our chips. We'll use the slogan, 'Bet you can't eat just one,' so kids make a game of eating as many as they can stuff in their mouth."

Mr. Junko, visualizing the stock getting fatter, adds, "Throw in a few vitamins. They're cheap. Then when the kid asks for Junkos, his health-conscious parent will agree."

"Fat idea!" Everyone applauds.

"Let's get started. What stuff do we put into our Junkos kids' line?" Mr. Junko inquires.

Miss Sweettaste, the company food tester, adds her mouthful. "Make them sweet. Every kid has a sweet tooth, you know."

CEO Junko gives a big belly laugh. "Sugar is cheap! Corn syrup is even cheaper!"

Miss Sweettaste continues. "Next, we've got to make our snacks oily. Kids like the mouth feel of oil."

Mr. Junko objects, "But food oils can be expensive! They also spoil quickly and shorten the shelf life of Junkos. A short shelf life means less profit."

Mr. Molecule, the food chemist, offers a solution. "First, we can use cheap oils, such as soy, corn, or cottonseed oils. Next, we can zap these oils with hydrogen. This produces partially hydrogenated oil. This process twists the fat molecules (known as trans fats) so the oil won't spoil. That will make it last longer on the shelf. It's legal, but not very healthy."

"What do you mean, not very healthy?" Mr. Junko asks.

Mrs. Lean, the company nutritionist, explains. "When you twist fat molecules to prolong the shelf life, the body doesn't recognize this as a natural food fat. Hydrogenated oils can cause fatty deposits to build up in arteries. There is also a general feeling among nutritionists that these factory fats could interfere with how well the body uses the more nutritious fats."

Mr. Junko inquires, "Does it make kids sick?"

Mrs. Lean responds, "Well . . . not right away."

Mr. Junko further inquires, "What do you mean?"

Mrs. Lean explains that these fake fats accumulate so slowly in the arteries that kids don't feel the bad effects for decades.

Mr. Junko asks, "Do we have to put these H-fats on the label that tells parents these fats are in our product? More parents are starting to read labels, you know."

Mr. Loophole, the company attorney, settles the case. "No problem," he reassures the group. "Due to a convenient label loophole, we don't have to list trans fats on the label. We can bury them in the total fat grams listing."

Mr. Junko concludes, "It's cheap and it's legal. Let's do it!" He adds, "Speaking of labels, what else should we put into Junkos?"

Mrs. Lean serves up her suggestions. "If we put in whole wheat, it will provide some fiber, and it's more nutritious."

Mr. Molecule objects. "Can't use whole wheat. It spoils sooner, it shortens the shelf life, and it's more expensive. But if we remove the bran and germ parts of the wheat, we can solve those problems."

Mr. Junko smiles, then asks, "So, how do we design a cute box that kids will like?"

Miss Labelle makes a contribution. "On the front of the box display a few healthy-sounding phrases, like *cholesterol free* and *natural.*"

Mrs. Lean is thinking, But all grains are cholesterol-free, and the word *natural* is misleading on labels. These words just make it look healthy.

Before she can speak up, the CEO turns to Mr. Costcutter, whose job it is to trim production costs.

"Puff it up," Mr. Costcutter advises. "Process it so that the food expands in volume and occupies more space in the box. The bread industry does this puffy trick all the time. That's why the big loaf of white bread doesn't weigh very much."

"Wow! I like that idea," Mr. Junko hollers, licking his fat cheeks and sensing more profit. "Air is cheap. And kids will have to eat more to fill up."

Mrs. Lean can't bite her tongue any longer. "Let me get this straight. We're operating under a sort of *more* for *less* principle—enticing kids to eat more Junkos while putting less nutrition into them."

"Welcome to the world of food marketing, Mrs. Lean," Mr. Junko says. "The bottom line is that junk food is cheaper to package than nutritious food, and kids can eat more of it before they feel full."

Mrs. Lean is thinking, If that's the bottom line that is so important here, no wonder kids have such big bottoms.

Mr. Junko winds up the meeting by reminding everyone of the company's mission statement. "Cheap to make, yet perceived by parents as healthy."

Fight the Food Industry

While you are trying to shape your children's tastes toward lean eating, advertisers are trying to convince kids that junk food is what they need. Children hear packaged foods are bad for them, but television advertising makes such food look cool and fun. Kids need their parents to set them straight. If you don't buy packaged foods, your kids will know you mean it when you say they shouldn't eat them. And so will the food industry. If you don't buy it, supermarkets won't stock it and food manufacturers won't make it. You can affect the offerings at fast-food chains as well. McDonald's McLean sandwich flopped because consumers didn't buy it. The buck stops and starts at home.

FAT DRINKS

Once upon a time kids drank milk and water. Nowadays they mostly drink sugar and corn syrup–sweetened beverages. It's not just a coincidence that the rising rate of childhood obesity over the past thirty years parallels the overconsumption of sweetened beverages. In fact, we believe that this is the prime contributor to the epidemic of childhood obesity. Because these beverages are less filling, children want to drink more. While milk is both satisfying and nutritious, making it hard to overdrink because its protein forms a filling curd in the stomach, kids can keep right on overdrinking sweet beverages. And the container sizes have gotten bigger as children's waists have gotten bigger—any correlation? Sweetened beverages are appropriately dubbed "empty calories" because not only do they provide little nutritional value, but the child's tummy feels empty soon afterward, so the child wants to drink more. Also, as you will learn on page 179, a metabolic quirk in corn syrup allows these calories to be easily deposited as excess fat. After thoroughly researching this topic, we have concluded that the single factor contributing most to the epidemic of childhood obesity is the overdrinking of corn syrup–sweetened beverages.

Get Rid of the Terrible Twos

Parents, could food technology be harming our children? Rid your home of the two foods I call the "terrible twos": corn syrup and hydrogenated oils. Foods containing these factory-made sugars and fats are the prime contributors to childhood obesity. For many children, simply omitting these two fake foods from their diet may be the most important change you can make to help them get lean.

FAT GENES

I think a second major cause of overfat kids is family eating habits. Many people assume that their kids are overweight because the genes they've inherited from the family make them fat.

Genes do not cause obesity. They can increase your child's chances of becoming overfat because some children inherit a *tendency* toward obesity. That means they inherit genes that promote fat storage. Usually, people carry such genes because their ancestors came from regions of the world that experienced famine for long periods of time. People who stored fat well survived better. Now their descendants are born with a predominance of fat-storing genes and still tend to store extra fat, even though they don't need it for survival. Children of this genetic type can remain lean, but they have to work harder at it.

In other words, a *tendency* is not the same thing as *destiny*. What's probably more important to children's future weight and health is that they also inherit their family's lifestyle and eating habits. If a lot of people in your family are overweight, don't assume that your child is doomed to be fat. It's not healthful (or accurate) for your kids to believe that they are born gainers. This feeling could be both a self-fulfilling and a self-defeating prophecy. You and your child should know that anyone can be lean if he eats and lives lean.

If your kids aren't living lean, it's not simply because of the genes they've inherited from you. They've also inherited habits, and I think these family habits have much more influence on your child's future health than genetics. Let's look at why.

Fat-eating parents have fat-eating children. Children inherit their parents' food preferences. Research shows that when one parent eats a lot of high-fat foods, the children are twice as likely to eat high-fat foods as are children whose parents eat low-fat foods. If both parents eat high-fat foods, their children are three to six times more likely to eat high-fat foods than are children of parents who eat low-fat diets. So, not only is it true that "you are what you eat," but "you are what your parents eat," too!

Genetically lean people, such as Asians, have a tendency to lose leanness when they move to our country and take up Western lifestyles and eating habits. Their genes certainly haven't changed, yet the way they live and eat has. Their experience illustrates for all of us the importance of nurture versus nature, or that your eating habits are more important than your genetic makeup in determining your weight. Most children are overfat not because of their genes, but because they eat the same food and have the same habits as their overfat parents.

Parents who move have kids who move. Like food preferences, exercise habits are also inherited from parents. Research shows that children who see their parents keeping up regular exercise programs are likely to follow their parents' example. When both parents are physically active, their children are six times more likely to be movers than if both parents are sedentary.

Children also tend to inherit their temperaments from their parents, and this too can have a great influence on their leanness. A person's temperament often determines how much of a mover she is. Jimmy and Johnny can eat the same amount of calories. Jimmy is a child with ants in

Lean Kids of Different Colors

There are racial differences in obesity trends. While the incidence of childhood obesity is climbing in American children of all races, African-American and Mexican-American children are getting fatter at faster rates than are other American children. The highest increase in obesity is among African-American girls.

There are many reasons for these racial differences in obesity. Studies show that there are metabolic differences in how children of different races burn calories. Caucasian girls tend to have a higher resting metabolic rate (RMR) than African-American girls. As a result, they burn more calories and tend to store less fat.

Until recently, not much attention was paid to these racial differences. It was thought that some cultures perceived leanness as attractive, others perceived fatness as attractive, and both were equally healthy. New insights into the long-term disease consequences of obesity have shown that this belief, while politically correct, is not scientifically correct.

Regardless of race, obesity is unhealthy. But a racially inherited tendency to store fat does not doom any child to obesity. Like all children, they can benefit from following the LEAN Kids Program.

his pants. He fidgets, paces, and is always on the go. His photographer father says, "There's no such thing as a still shot for my son." Johnny, on the other hand, is a sitter. He likes to veg out in front of the TV or sit on the sidelines playing his Game Boy while the rest of the kids are playing soccer. One temperament type is not better than another. Kids are just different. But Johnny the sitter is at a higher risk for obesity than Jimmy the mover.

While temperament, parental lifestyles, and eating habits have the greatest influence on a child's becoming overfat, the encouraging news is that parental habits can also greatly influence a child in becoming lean. When parents stay or become lean, their children are more likely to stay or become lean, too. The bottom line: Fat parents tend to have fat kids, and lean parents tend to have lean children.

If you're still skeptical about the idea that your family habits are more important to your weight and health than are genes, consider this: The rapid increase in obesity in recent years happened too fast to be blamed on genes.

How Kids Get Underfit and Out of Shape

When our fitness advisor, Sean Foy, was nineteen, he suffered a severe knee injury that required surgery, and he wore a full-leg plaster cast for eight weeks. The worst part about wearing the cast for that long was not just his inability to move, but also the itchiness of the injured leg. As the weeks passed, a strange thing happened. He noticed by the second week of wearing the cast that he could scratch the top of his thigh with his fingers. By the fourth week, he could scratch his knee! By the eighth week, he could almost touch his calf.

When the doctor took the cast off, Sean was shocked to find how much his leg had shriveled in only eight weeks of inactivity. Then he realized that while he had a nineteen-year-old body, he now had a ninety-nine-year-old leg. He couldn't stand on it, couldn't bend it, couldn't move it. In just eight weeks, Sean's leg had aged physiologically eighty years. That's just one illustration of the fact that inactivity can cause us to lose muscle at any age.

The body was made to move. For adults and children, not using our muscles enough accelerates the deterioration of the body. And the problem is that our children are living in a world that makes it easy to be inactive. Let's look at some of the other causes of our children's increasing inactivity.

FAT SCHOOLS

Lunches are high-fat and high-sugar; vending machines serve syrupy drinks and snacks. Those are the health lessons kids are learning at school.

While the United States government has continued to emphasize the importance of physical education, in many schools these programs have been reduced to a minor consideration or excluded altogether. Consider the following national trends in physical education:

- According to the President's Council on Physical Fitness and Sports (PCPFS), some students get as little as one hour of physical education a week.
- According to 2001 data from the Centers for Disease Control, the majority of kids of all ages do not get enough physical activity. The CDC considers lack of physical fitness a serious public health problem.
- According to the School Health Policies Programs Study (SHPPS), only 8.0 percent of elementary schools, 6.4 percent of middle/junior high schools, and 5.8 percent of senior high schools provide daily physical education or its equivalent for the entire school year for students in all grades.

Why, with the overwhelming evidence supporting the health benefits of physical activity, do we continue to see enrollment in physical education classes decline? Well, primarily because our schools have less money. In addition, they're increasingly pressured to quantify success in reading, writing, and arithmetic. While schools emphasize the 3 R's, *running* is not one of them.

Dr. David Satcher, the U.S. Surgeon General from 1998 to 2002, called physical inactivity a "major epidemic" in the United States, stating, "I think we've made a serious error by not requiring physical education in grades K through 12. We are paying a tremendous price for this physical inactivity. People pay with pain and suffering, and society pays with money and lost productivity."

FAT SITTING

American kids spend more time sitting and watching a screen than running and playing (and sometimes more time than they spend in the classroom). A 1999 national survey found that kids aged two to eighteen spend, on average, over four hours a day watching television, watching videotapes, playing video games, or using a computer. Most of this time (two hours and forty-six minutes per day) is spent watching television. One-third of children and adolescents watch television for more than three hours a day, and nearly one-fifth (17 percent) watch more than five hours of television a day. Since there aren't any ads promoting fresh fruits and veggies, kids see only ads for high-sugar and high-fat junk foods, often hawked by a sports-star role model. Kids naturally then perceive this food as the norm and assume, "This is what everyone eats."

It's no coincidence that over the past thirty years, as technology, television viewing, and computer game playing for kids has increased, so too has the prevalence of childhood obesity and diabetes.

PARENTS ARE AFRAID

Once upon a time kids were lean. They ran, rode, hopped, skipped down sidewalks, gathered for games in neighborhood parks, and walked or biked to and from school. Those were kids on the move. Nowadays, suburban neighborhoods no longer have sidewalks. The fear of child molestation and abduction requires parents to fearfully shadow their kids. Kids are driven or bused to school. Parents feel safer with their kids staying home (often sitting in front of a TV). Neighborhood playgrounds and recreation centers, if they still exist, are off limits. Modern living

Scary Screen Stats

- Research shows that children's resting metabolic rates (how many calories they burn) decrease between 12 and 16 percent when they "zone out" on the tube.
- The amount of time spent watching TV directly correlates with kids requesting and parents purchasing foods high in sugar and fat.
- Parents frequently underestimate the amount of time children spend watching television or playing computer games.
- Parents are often unaware of what their kids eat while they watch.
- Children who watch more TV tend to eat a higher percentage of fat in their diets.
- The increase of overweight children is directly related to the increase in time spent watching television or videos.
- Studies show that the more TV children watch, the higher their cholesterol is likely to be, and the more obese they are likely to become.
- Because of the fat messages children are getting from the media, the American Academy of Pediatrics has recently advised pediatricians to take a "media history" during a school-age child's regular checkup.

promotes fatness, not leanness. Is it any wonder that we now have a generation of indoor kids who put on extra pounds because they have more opportunities to sit than move?

PARENTS ARE POOPED

Do you ever feel hurried, stressed, anxious, overextended, exhausted, burnt out, or overwhelmed by the pace of living? If you answer yes, you're not alone. For many of us, our schedules have become as overloaded as our bodies. When we asked parents what the greatest barrier to maintaining a consistent fitness program was for them, nearly all answered *time* and *energy*.

We have less time to play catch or kick a ball with our kids, less time to go for after-dinner walks. We don't even have time to supervise our kids when they play outside, and we don't feel that they're safe if they go out on their own. We have less energy for investing in one of our family's greatest assets: health and fitness. Unless you make health a passionate priority, you cannot hope to overcome this challenge. Yet it is possible. Your determination will make the difference. The LEAN Kids Program will show you how.

How Kids Get Unhappy

Unhappiness is the third major risk to our children in their school-age years. More and more children are in therapy or even taking medication to address their feelings of discontent. And the range of conditions they suffer from is broad—from moodiness to serious depression and suicidal tendencies. So the first thing I need to clarify is that this is not a book about the mental health of school-aged children, nor is the LEAN Kids Program designed to address serious mental illness. If your child is extremely depressed or suffers from an eating disorder such as anorexia or bulimia, you need to consult your pediatrician and/or a therapist.

However, short of those serious disease conditions of the mind, there are a lot of unhappy kids out there. There are kids who don't like their bodies. There are kids who are depressed because they're always chosen last for team sports. There are kids who feel different, and to a child that means feeling bad. These are the children the LEAN Kids Program can help.

TOO MUCH TEASING

The three greatest risks to our children's health travel in a pack—wherever you find Mr. Overfat and Ms. Underfit, you usually find Miss Unhappiness not far behind!

One of the leading causes of unhappiness in school-age children is overfatness and underfitness. Overfat kids are teased by their friends.

Underfit kids have less fun at recess. Whatever makes your child feel left out or different makes him feel sad.

Even children who start out lean can end up overfat if unhappiness leads them there. Sadness in children can be caused by a variety of factors, but the predominant one in my view is stress.

AMERICAN KIDS ARE BECOMING STRESSED

Stress is the way we react physically, mentally, and emotionally to various conditions, changes, and demands in our lives. Scientists tell us that just the right amount of stress is good for the body. Managed stress, like managed weight, is healthy. Good stress makes life interesting, prevents boredom, and challenges us to grow and change. Bad stress, however, can make you sick—and fat. The stress response is like a drug. The right dose in the right situation helps, but an overdose can be harmful.

When good stress keeps you interested, challenged, and productive in response to situations that threaten your well-being, we call it a *biochemical turn-on*. We call stress bad when it is chronic, unresolved, and unproductive, and when it shuts down the brain's natural neurostimulants. We call this kind of stress response a *biochemical turn-off*.

Stress increases chance of illness. You can worry yourself sick! Excessive and unmanaged stress can weaken the immune system. Studies have shown a direct link between the nervous system and the immune system, so what affects one affects the other.

Stress promotes fat storage. During periods of high stress, a child may ignore internal satiety signals and keep right on eating. This is dubbed the "stew and chew" response—eating to relieve stress. The stress hormone, cortisol, stimulates insulin, which promotes fat storage, especially around the waist, dubbed "stress fat." Stress can trigger carbohydrate cravings, remembered by the classic connection: *stressed* spelled backward is *desserts*.

Stress impairs sound sleep. High levels of stress hormones can impair sleep. As a result, the young student can't learn as well the next day. Irritability often leads to conflict, and more stress.

Stress can lead to depression. Stress interferes with the normal function of "happy hormones" and can lead to depression.

The Carry-Over Effect

Just as overfatness, underfitness, and unhappiness tend to occur together, so is the reverse true. Healthy and strong kids tend to be happier. One of the perks of the LEAN Kids Program is that once your
children are eating, moving, and feeling healthier, they will tend to
make healthier choices in all areas of life—including saying no to
drugs, smoking, alcohol, and other harmful practices because they
like themselves.

Questions You May Have

Now that you have a thorough understanding of the causes of overfatness, underfitness, and unhappiness, you'll be glad to know that the
LEAN Kids Program was specifically designed to reverse these trends. In
the next chapter, you'll see how the LEAN Kids Program does that.

First, I'd like to address the questions I hear most frequently in my
office concerning weight control.

I'VE TRIED LOTS OF DIETS AND THE EXTRA FAT IS SO HARD TO LOSE. WHY?

The body fights fat loss. Once upon a time people had to hunt, fish, and
forage for food. Our species developed in an age of feast or famine. The
hungry human body adapted to this erratic food supply by developing
the ability to store body fat for fuel during times of famine.

Today there's a food store on every American corner, and most people
in the United States have to deal with food excess, not shortage. Yet we're
still armed with our fat-storing survival genes. The body doesn't give up
millions of years of genetic programming in a mere hundred years,
which is why crash diets don't work.

The body perceives any sudden drastic changes in food consumption—such as crash dieting—as life-threatening. It automatically, and protectively, resets its resting metabolic rate to burn fewer calories and hold on to its stored fat.

There are two ways for the mind to fool the body and avoid this fat-saving response. One is to trick the body by *gradually* lessening food-calorie consumption so the body doesn't perceive that you're really eating less. It's as if the mind doesn't let the body know it's on a diet. The mind sneaks in a new way of eating without alarming the body into resetting its fat-storage gauge. The second, and better, way to trick the body is to start eating *lean* foods—lower-calorie foods that are filling without being fattening. Because the body doesn't get hungry, it doesn't fight this new way of eating.

Adding exercise to your new eating habits is the most effective way to lose weight. If you maintain the same level of food consumption but burn more calories, your body won't click into starvation mode and you'll see the pounds melt away.

MY EIGHT-YEAR-OLD IS OVERFAT, YET HE DOESN'T SEEM TO EAT MORE THAN HIS LEAN SISTER. COULD IT BE HIS METABOLISM?

Yes. Some kids have a fast metabolism and are born calorie burners. Others have a slower metabolism and burn fat more slowly. Whether your child is a fat-burner or a storer depends on an inherited trait. "Storers" need to make healthier choices, yet they can overcome their slower metabolism to become lean, too.

OUR CHILD HAS TROUBLE KEEPING EXCESS WEIGHT OFF. COULD IT BE HER THYROID?

This is a question I'm frequently asked during obesity counseling, and the answer is almost always no. Endocrine problems, such as a low thyroid (or "hypothyroid"), are a cause of obesity in less than *1 percent* of children. So it's very unlikely that this is really your child's problem. Yet just to be sure, look for these clues to an endocrine problem:

Heavy but short children may have an endocrine cause

of obesity. If a child is overfat but under-height (much heavier than average, yet much shorter than average on the growth charts), suspect an endocrine problem. Children with endocrine problems tend to be short.

Heavy but tall or average-height children do not have an endocrine cause of obesity. Most overfat-from-being-overfed children are big, in both height and weight. They usually plot near the top of the growth chart in weight and height.

HOW CAN I KEEP MY CHILD FROM GETTING ANOREXIA OR BULIMIA? I DON'T WANT HER TO BE OBSESSED WITH HER WEIGHT.

Right on! Children develop eating disorders as a way to control something in their life when everything seems out of control. This concern is why I constantly stress the word *lean* (meaning the right weight and muscle development for a child's body type) rather than using words like "thin" or even "trim," which call too much attention to a child's looks and have little to do with the child's state of health. The LEAN Kids Program is designed to address the child's weight, strength, and feelings. It is intentionally not a calorie-counting, menu-planned, weight-loss program because those kinds of restrictive eating plans tend to throw a person's emotional relationship with food out of balance. Denying your child certain foods (or enough food) can lead to cravings and inevitable bingeing—which your child then feels regretful and even shameful about. That's an unhealthy and unhappy cycle that the LEAN Kids Program is carefully designed to avoid.

Yet if you feel your child is particularly susceptible to these kinds of feelings, you might want to keep the following advice in mind:

Address her weight very little. When I monitor kids on the program in my office, I seldom mention the "W" word. Sometimes I weigh sensitive kids only every *other* visit. Instead, I focus on their feelings. "How's your energy?" "Do you like the new whole-wheat bread your mom is giving you?" "How'd you do in the last soccer game? Was it fun to have more energy?"

Scale down! Don't obsess about weighing your child. Leave that up to your child's doctor. Scale watching is unnecessary for a growing child and calls too much attention to the weight. For children, excessive weight watching sets them up for eating disorders. They worry if they weigh too much and often overcompensate with undernutrition.

And the truth is that you don't want your child to *lose* weight. You want your overfat child to maintain his current weight until he leans out. You should trust that if you are wholeheartedly following the LEAN Kids Program, your child's weight will take care of itself.

OUR FIRST CHILD IS VERY OVERWEIGHT. I'M EXPECTING A SECOND BABY. WHAT CAN I DO TO HELP MY NEW BABY GROW UP LEAN?

Rewind the tape of your first child and ask yourself where you could have made better health choices. Here's a checklist you can use to build a little lean body from birth:

Breast-feed your baby. Breast-feeding lowers the risk of obesity, and the longer the infant is breast-fed, the lower the risk. During breast-feeding an infant learns to say yes and no to food by sucking at the breast. As soon as he's full and satisfied, he stops eating. He may continue to comfort suck awhile, but the breast naturally offers low-calorie milk at this point in the nursing cycle. And there is certainly no push by mommy to "finish the breast."

On the other hand, the bottle-fed baby often gets pushed to finish the bottle. And he can easily get excess milk (and excess calories) from simply comfort sucking because the milk the bottle offers at the end of his eating cycle is just as rich as the milk he started with. This child can grow up to become oblivious to his satiety signals, or his *satiety set point* (when the infant feels full) may be reset upward.

Delay solid foods. The longer you can wait to feed your child solids, the better. Try to breast-feed your baby exclusively for at least the first six months of her life. When you do begin solids, introduce your baby to nutrient-dense foods (those that pack a lot of nutrition per calorie) as opposed to calorie-dense foods (those that pack a lot of calories in a small volume). For example, start with veggies instead of fruits; fruits instead of juice; water diluted with 100 percent fruit juice rather than juice drinks.

Shape young tastes early. Make your own baby food rather than serving jarred or canned foods. That way your baby is programmed to regard the taste of homemade foods as the norm. Most important, limit sweetened beverages.

Offer smaller portions. Respect that tiny children have tiny tummies, about the size of their fist. Never serve them more than that at one time. Give them more only if they ask you for it.

A FRIEND OF MINE TOLD ME THAT THERE ARE CERTAIN "HIGH RISK" YEARS FOR WEIGHT GAIN. IS THAT TRUE?

Yes, it certainly is—and too few parents are aware of it. Here's what you need to know.

During pregnancy. If Mom overfeeds herself during the prenatal period, she can produce an excess of fat cells to grow in her baby and therefore lead to an obese newborn. The last trimester of pregnancy is the riskiest, since that's the time when the number of fat cells in the newborn greatly increases.

Infancy (birth to two years). The next critical period is from birth to two years, during which breast-fed and formula-fed babies have different risk patterns for developing later obesity. So do infants who are given homemade food versus store-bought food. If you are bottle-feeding, you will have to make a special effort to avoid overfeeding your child. And if you must rely on packaged baby foods, be aware that you will make lean living more of a challenge for your child in years to come.

Middle childhood (five to nine years): This is another period of rapid growth during which both the size and the number of fat cells in the body increases. This is when lean eating is most important.

Adolescence. During the early teen years, fat is redistributed throughout the body as the child's body matures. During this period, an increase in abdominal fat is an especially high risk.

4

HOW THE LEAN KIDS PROGRAM WORKS

Puts Child in Biochemical Balance

Now that we've looked carefully at the causes of our weight, fitness, and happiness problems, we're ready to talk in more detail about how the LEAN Kids Program works to help children in all three areas.

The reason kids are getting sicker, sadder, and fatter is because their growing bodies are out of biochemical balance. The body is often described as a "chemical soup." If the hormones and other biochemicals are in the right balance, the body is healthful and happy. If not, we can feel sick, sad, and fat. The LEAN Kids Program's four pillars—lifestyle, exercise, attitude, and nutrition—all work together as a health maintenance plan to keep the child biochemically balanced.

In this chapter, we'll look at the role of hormones in your child's health and why keeping them in balance is so important, and we'll review how the LEAN Kids Program acts to help maintain that balance.

Promotes Hormonal Harmony

The biochemical basis of the LEAN Kids Program is to put the child's body—and brain—in *hormonal harmony*. Hormones are chemical messengers that travel throughout the body, telling the organs how to work together. They work best when they are at just the right levels—not too much, and not too little. The LEAN Kids Program helps hormones stay at their best levels.

Think of each hormone as an instrument in an orchestra and the LEAN Kids Program as the conductor. If too many hormones are released at the wrong time, like the percussion section of an orchestra coming on too strong too soon, the whole body gets out of balance, becoming too fat or too skinny, too hyper or too tired. By instructing children to live lean, the conductor brings each instrument in the orchestra into harmony, and beautiful music—or wellness—results.

All of the hormones I discuss below are intimately related to and affected by the LEAN Kids Program. All are produced and affected by the eating and exercising cycles of the body. For good health, all these hormones must be kept in balance, and that is what living the LEAN Kids Program way will do for your children. Let's look at each of the hormones affected by the LEAN Kids Program individually so you can see how the plan works to improve your child's health.

While there are hundreds of hormones trying to work in harmony throughout the body, there are two main groups that are influenced most by the LEAN Kids Program: grow-right hormones, and feel-right hormones.

GROW-RIGHT HORMONES

There are several different hormones in the body that I consider grow-right hormones. Let's look at them one by one.

Growth hormone (GH) helps your child grow just right, as the name implies. Secreted by the pituitary (the grape-size gland near the base of the brain), GH helps the cells of each organ grow by instructing them how to use nutrients in food for energy. GH helps build muscle, for example, by telling the muscle cells to take up the amino acids from the foods that enter the blood and assemble them together as muscle-building proteins. GH tells the fat cells to release some of their stored fat for energy when the other cells need that fuel to grow. Children with GH deficiency tend to be short and fat because their cells are lacking these crucial instructions.

"So how do I help my child get the right amount of growth hormone?" you may wonder. Read on to see why the LEAN Kids Program takes care of the problem for you.

- **Restful sleep manufactures growth hormone.** Growth hormone is produced naturally in the body, particularly at night during deep or slow wave sleep. The LEAN Kids Program promotes a restful night's sleep by encouraging plenty of exercise during the day and making sure that dinner is a meal that sits comfortably in your child's stomach.
- **Strenuous exercise is a potent, natural stimulator of growth hormone.** Dubbed the "youth hormone," GH peaks after puberty and goes downhill from then on. It's unfair but true that as we age we produce less GH, but we continue to need it. Both kids and adults can get more of the benefits of this great hormone by increasing their levels of exercise. After adolescence, GH functions primarily to help the body provide energy for repair and maintenance, and GH could more correctly be called the "maintenance hormone." One of the reasons we tend to get fatter as we get older is because diminishing GH causes the body to store excess fat. Since GH increases muscle and decreases body fat—two main goals of the LEAN Kids Program—GH could be called the "leaning out" hormone.

Insulin is a key grow-right hormone. After growth hormone, the next grow-right hormone is *insulin.* Insulin is one of the body's most important chemical messengers for a variety of reasons (and you'll hear more about them throughout this book), but one of its critical jobs is to help regulate growth. Insulin is a good example of the necessity of hormonal balance: Too much insulin and you get tired and fat, too little and you get weak and sick. Just the right dose and you grow and feel just right. That's why keeping insulin in proper balance is so important for children.

FEEL-RIGHT AND THINK-RIGHT HORMONES

One of the goals of the LEAN Kids Program is not only to have a healthy child, but also to have a happy one. The happy hormones, which include serotonin, neuropeptide Y, galanin, and endorphins, mostly affect emotions and other brain functions. They are all involved in the eating and

Avoid Too Much of a Good Thing

Children who have just the right amount of grow-right hormones are likely to grow optimally, meaning children will reach their genetically programmed height and have just the right amount of body fat for their body type. Resist the temptation of advertisers who promote GH supplements as weight-loss tools. While GH injections have been proven safe and effective in helping GH-deficient children, we don't know if they are safe for other uses. There is a flurry of research being conducted to determine if GH is as safe and effective as a fat-loss or muscle-building supplement. Preliminary studies suggest that it is not, certainly not for kids.

exercising cycles of the body, and hence their function in your child's body is improved by the LEAN Kids Program.

Serotonin increases well-being. Known as a feel-good or calming hormone, serotonin is a hormone the body craves in just the right amounts. Too much and a person could become anxious or silly, too little and a person could become sad and depressed. The body and brain get used to the right level of this mood elevator and can even begin to depend on it for a sense of well-being.

What happens to carbohydrate cravers is that they get too dependent on the good feelings of serotonin. Refined carbohydrates (like white bread and pasta) and sugary sweets trigger serotonin release. A carb craver learns that eating this way makes him feel better, but the feelings don't last long, and when they wear off the cravings begin anew.

Let's revisit our friends Fat Freddie and Lean Lucy. Over time, Freddy makes the food-mood connection between eating sweets and feeling good. Lucy, on the other hand, after years of lean living and eating, has different craving chemistries. Her food-mood connection is not as dependent on junk foods. Rather, her body is used to the levels brought on by her lean eating and living. She never craves the artificially high spikes in serotonin levels brought on by sweet carb consumption. Because she's a mover and her exercise stimulates happy hormones, she doesn't depend on sweets for a good mood. In fact, during a birthday party when she occasionally indulges in a second piece of junk cake, her serotonin levels may overreact, causing her to feel "yucky."

Endorphins are the happy hormones. Endorphins (named for *endo*genous m*orphins*) are nicknamed the happy hormones because they are the brain's natural narcotics. You've probably heard that exercise releases endorphins; that's why movers continually crave exercise. It's certainly better for them than craving carbs! Endorphins are kept at healthy levels by the emphasis on moving in the LEAN Kids Program.

Neuropeptide Y (NPY) craves carbohydrates. Carbohydrates are the body's prime source of energy, especially for the brain. When the body runs out of carbs, it craves more. NPY's job is to be sure the body and the brain get enough healthy carbs for energy. As children use up their stores of energy, their blood sugar dips and triggers the release of NPY, which triggers the brain to crave more carbs.

This is one of the reasons why children crave more carbs if they skip breakfast or go without eating for a long time. NPY may be the neurochemical reason why most of us prefer a high-carbohydrate breakfast after using up carb stores during the night. In fact, NPY tends to be highest in the morning, which makes sense, as if it's telling the body to restock its store of carbs for energy to get the brain and body going.

NPY is kept at healthful levels by the complex carbohydrates in the LEAN Kids Program.

Galanin is the fat-craving hormone. Just as NPY rises when carbs are low, galanin is the body's internal messenger that prompts the child to eat more fat when the fat stores are low. This fat-craving neurochemical tends to be highest in the evening, when the smart body knows it needs to store fat for the sleeping, overnight fast. That's just one of the reasons the LEAN Kids Program emphasizes a right-fat, not a low-fat, diet. Eating the right fats will keep galanin at healthful levels.

Cortisol is the stress hormone. The stress hormone cortisol is like the other hormones: Too much or too little is bad, but just the right amount keeps us alert and responsive. Cortisol also helps regulate appetite, control body fat, and maintain mental functioning. It can act like a rescue hormone by squeezing sugar out of your liver to fuel your brain when you don't have any other energy sources available. Yet high levels of cortisol put your body in a state of stress and make you feel irritable. Your child will benefit on many levels from the way the LEAN Kids Program keeps cortisol in balance.

Changes Young Cravings

One way the LEAN Kids Program helps the child's body regain biochemical balance is to curb cravings by keeping hormones at the right levels at the right times of the day. Cravings and binge eating are often caused by a hormonal imbalance. Take, for example, the child who skips breakfast. After the long night the body is low on energy and craves carbs. When a child skips breakfast, those cravings build and build and can prompt the body to overeat later in the day. The high level of carbs ingested during this binge meal cause an insulin surge, which prompts the body to overeat again. The cycle of cravings and out-of-balance hormones has begun.

Cravings are the body's natural, defensive response to nutritional deficiencies. It's the body's way of saying, "Hey, I need something right now!" The problem with cravings is that when they are a response to unhealthful eating (like skipping breakfast), they lead us to crave unhealthy things (like bingeing on carbs). That bingeing, in turn, throws our hormones out of balance—which leads to more unhealthful cravings, and the cycle is renewed.

You can see how easily our natural Wisdom of the Body is corrupted. One mistake leads to another until our body forgets the way it is supposed to eat and supposed to feel. That's why the LEAN Kids Program puts so much emphasis on regaining the Wisdom of the Body, or reteaching the body to crave the kind of healthy eating that keeps our hormones in balance.

Let's look at how the LEAN Kids Program puts the child on crave control.

EATING HEALTHFULLY CURBS CRAVINGS

If unhealthful eating leads to the cravings that result in binge eating and throw our hormones out of balance, then you can see how healthful eating alone can go a long way in reversing this pattern. If you eat nutritious foods in the right amounts and at the right times of day, your body won't build up cravings that lead you to binge. You'll eat just the right amount to keep your hormones in balance, so you also will avoid the hormonal surges that can also lead to unhealthful cravings. According to the Wisdom of the Body principle, the body should crave what's good for it and shun what's bad for it. The goal of the LEAN Kids Program is to protect the child's natural Wisdom of the Body by changing her cravings—to crave what is healthy and shun what is unhealthy. If your Wisdom of the Body is broken, the secret to fixing it is more healthful eating. Yet that's the very thing you've forgotten how to do. How do you remember?

GRAZING CURBS CRAVINGS

One of the first and easiest steps to take is to start grazing. On the LEAN Kids Program, I encourage parents to let kids graze—eat small, nutritious meals throughout the day. These small meals help to keep children's bodies in biochemical balance and their hormones at just the right levels. When you eat a steady and varied diet of healthy foods, your body secretes just the right balance of hormones that give you a feeling of well-being. Children who learn this good feeling at an early age instinctively

---

Run Away from Your Cravings

Exercise helps kids curb cravings. When you run away from that doughnut, the endorphins or feel-good hormones that are released during the strenuous exercise help overcome the craving. When your child craves an unhealthful treat, try distracting her by suggesting, "Go outside and play for a while."

want good foods that keep these hormones in balance (see Encourage Good Grazing, page 215).

LEAN EATING GIVES GOOD GUT FEELINGS

The good feeling from healthful eating is one of the best medicines for a child who has lost her natural Wisdom of the Body. Persons on the LEAN Kids Program call it a "good gut feeling." Children like feeling good! As they live on the LEAN Kids Program, they'll notice a yucky feeling that super-sugary snacks give them. Yet they'll notice that they feel alert, satisfied, and calm after meals. And it won't be hard for you to talk them into eating in a way that helps them feel that way again soon. I've found children on the LEAN Kids Program quickly make the connection between good eating and good feelings.

LEAN KIDS SAY

"If I eat something that is too junky, I feel sick
to my stomach and have stinky poop."
—JACOB, AGE NINE

HEALTHFUL FOOD SHAPES YOUNG TASTES

Kids will choose taste over nutrition, unless they are programmed otherwise. One of the ways the LEAN Kids Program fights unhealthy cravings is by working to shape young tastes so that kids don't like eating the kinds of foods that can lead to the craving-bingeing cycle. From six to twelve years is a window of opportunity when children's taste buds can be programmed toward healthy taste preferences. The LEAN Kids Program is designed to maximize that opportunity.

Children form lifelong eating habits in the school years. A child who grows up nourished with wholesome, fresh foods will learn to prefer these foods the rest of her life because she develops that taste. These flavors become her norm, and if she tries oversweet, high-fat, processed foods only rarely, they will taste odd to her. By not just exposing but immersing your children in a diet of whole, fresh, healthful and homemade foods, you can give them the kind of expectations that will protect their health for life.

Living the LEAN Kids Program

Now that you have a better understanding of why hormones are so critical to our overall health and how the LEAN Kids Program works to keep them in balance, we're hoping that you're eager to make lean living a part of your life. Let's get started in the next chapter, where we'll show you how to make an assessment of your child's weight and fitness so you can personalize the LEAN Kids Program for your child and your family.

PART TWO

HOW TO USE THE LEAN KIDS PROGRAM

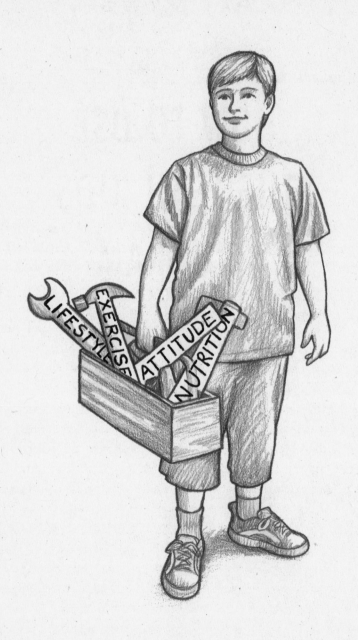

5

GETTING STARTED

Assess Your Child

In the first part of this book, we reviewed the three biggest risks to the health of our school-age children—overfatness, underfitness, and unhappiness. We looked at what was causing these problems in epidemic proportions, and we reviewed how the LEAN Kids Program works to combat them. Before you can get started with the LEAN Kids Program and begin following the plan's lifestyle, exercise, attitude, and nutritional advice, you first need to determine where your child is on the health scale. Is he overfat? Is she underweight? Is your presently lean child at risk of becoming overfat?

Sometimes it's obvious that a child is overfat, but for many parents it's actually difficult to tell. For instance, a big child may weigh a lot and be larger than his peers without being overfat. On the other hand, preteen girls may already be emulating media images of the overthin set and want to diet when there is no need. That's why parents need to know if and how much their child is overfat, or in some cases underweight, in order to gauge how much of the LEAN Kids Program their child needs.

What's important to know is that a child's leanness (and an adult's, for that matter) is not just a question of how much he weighs. In order to assess the balance of fat and muscle on your child's skeletal frame, you need to take several factors into account: what the scale and growth charts reveal; the fat folds your fingers feel; the body your eyes see; what risks factors affect your child; and what your child's doctor ultimately decides. Follow these four steps.

Step 1: Understand the Growth Charts

You bring your seven-year-old to the doctor for her yearly checkup. The nurse plots her weight and height on a standard growth chart. Near the end of the visit, the doctor pronounces, "According to the charts, your child is about ten pounds overweight. She is in the 50th percentile in height, yet she is in the 85th for weight, and her BMI is 18.3." You never thought of your child as fat. And perhaps you don't know what these numbers mean, or what you should do about them. Before you begin the assessment of your child's physical growth and fitness level, let's go inside the numbers and see what they mean and how they apply to most children, and especially to *your* child.

GROWTH CHARTS MADE SIMPLE

Growth charts are what your child's healthcare provider uses to plot your child's height and weight at annual checkups. Before you chart your child's physical growth at home, here are some important facts you should know about using and interpreting the charts:

- Growth charts are compiled from *average* measurements of thousands of children of both genders, across all areas of the United States, and including all racial backgrounds. Because of this diversity of sampling, the numbers may not accurately reflect your child's optimal growth. Growth charts are simply screening tools, nothing more. They give a *clue* to a possible growth concern, not a diagnosis.
- Growth charts are divided into percentile lines (see sample charts on pages 63 and 64). The term "percentile" means where your child fits into the group. For instance, the 50th percentile is an average, which means that out of a hundred children, fifty weigh more than your child and fifty weigh less. The 85th percentile means that 15 percent of kids weigh more than your child, and 85 percent weigh less.
- The higher the weight percentile, the more risky it is. A child at

or above the 95th weight percentile would be considered at risk of being or becoming overfat, regardless of the height percentile.

- The greater the difference between the weight percentile and the height percentile, the greater your concern should be. For example, the child who plots in the 80th percentile for weight and the 50th percentile for height would be more of a concern than a child who plots around the 50th percentile for both height and weight.
- The year-to-year trend is more useful than the actual numbers.

BMI (BODY MASS INDEX) CHARTS MADE SIMPLE

The BMI is a more accurate chart for predicting the risk for being overfat. Also, unlike the standard height and weight charts mentioned above, the BMI charts can predict health risks. BMI charts reflect children's weight relative to their height. These charts are helpful in tracking a person's growth from two years of age throughout adulthood. Here's what you should know about the numbers:

- A BMI at or greater than 95 percent classifies the child as "overweight" and at the highest risk of being obese and developing health problems related to obesity.
- Between the 85th and 95th percentiles, the child is classified as "at risk" of being overweight. Between the 5th and 85th percentiles is considered the "normal" zone.
- Less than the 5th percentile, the child could be "underweight," or the child could be genetically petite or a healthy, lean child.
- You will notice that the lines on the BMI chart progressively dip for the period from two to six years, during which time children go through a leaning-out stage of growing faster in height than in weight. Then the opposite occurs, and children gain more weight (both fat and muscle) relative to their height, and the curve starts going up. The year at which the line on the curve starts going up is called the *adiposity rebound*, which for the average child is around six years of age. The earlier a child goes

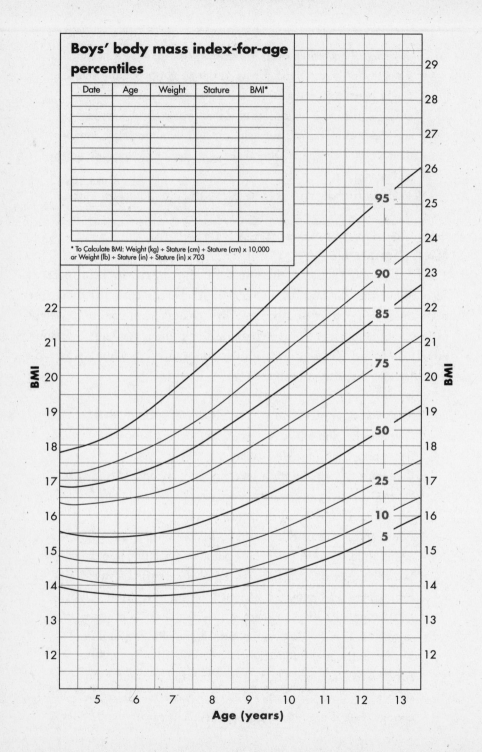

Boys' body mass index-for-age percentiles

Date	Age	Weight	Stature	BMI*

* To Calculate BMI: Weight (kg) ÷ Stature (cm) ÷ Stature (cm) x 10,000
or Weight (lb) ÷ Stature (in) ÷ Stature (in) x 703

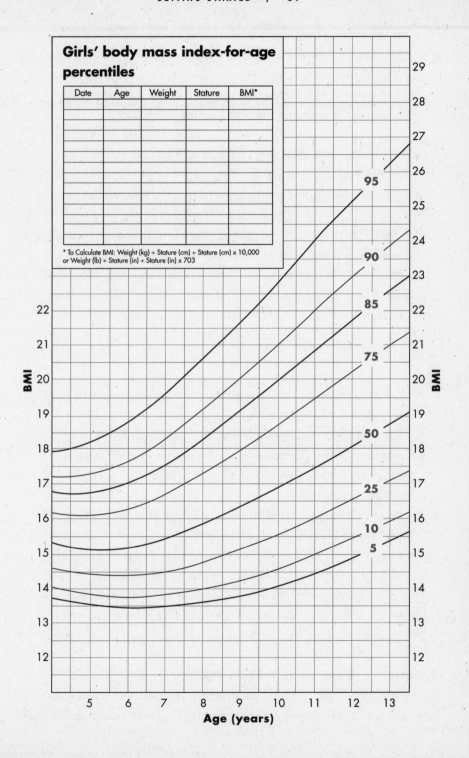

Girls' body mass index-for-age percentiles

Date	Age	Weight	Stature	BMI*

* To Calculate BMI: Weight (kg) ÷ Stature (cm) ÷ Stature (cm) x 10,000
or Weight (lb) ÷ Stature (in) ÷ Stature (in) x 703

through this adiposity rebound, the higher the risk of the child becoming overfat. You will notice that a child with a BMI in the 95th percentile starts the rebound between four and five years of age, a year or two earlier than the child in the 50th percentile. This child is at greater risk of becoming overfat.

HEALTH CONSIDERATIONS OF THE 95TH PERCENTILE

If your child's weight and/or BMI are in the 95th percentile, it does not always mean that your child is obese. However, it is a *red flag* that your child may be at risk of becoming obese and having more health problems, depending on the other factors listed on page 78. Or the child could just be big and muscular. The situation isn't clear-cut, so researchers have measured the body fat of children with a weight and BMI in the "overweight" range to see what these numbers mean. The findings, listed below, indicate that these children are at greater risk than others:

- A BMI at or above the 95th percentile is associated with a higher risk of the child's having high blood pressure, elevated blood lipids, and elevated insulin levels during childhood.
- Sixty percent of children with a BMI greater than the 95th percentile have at least one of the above three risk factors for cardiovascular disease.
- Ninety-five percent of children with a BMI at or above the 95th percentile tend to carry excess body fat.
- Five of six children whose BMI was in the "normal" range (6th to 84th percentiles) did not have an increased percentage of body fat (as scientifically measured). Only one out of four children whose BMI was in the "obese" range had a percentage of body fat in the "normal" range.

LOOK AT THE BIG PICTURE

The most important thing to remember when you're reading growth charts is that they are just screening tools. The percentile number they

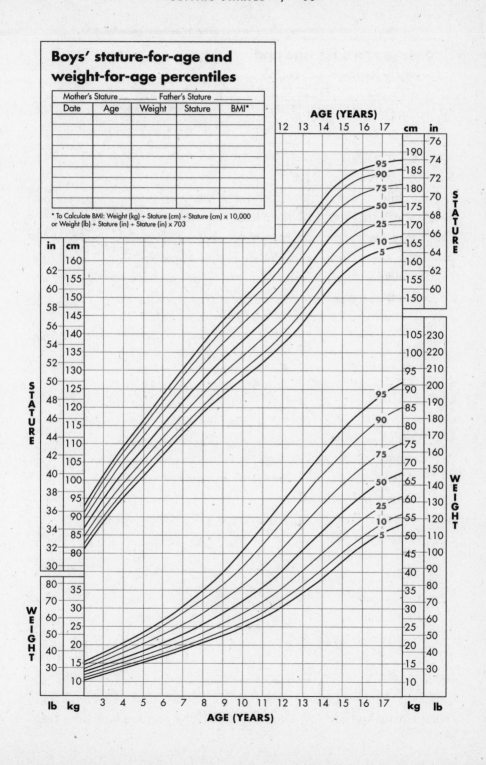

Boys' stature-for-age and weight-for-age percentiles

Mother's Stature _____ Father's Stature _____

Date	Age	Weight	Stature	BMI*

* To Calculate BMI: Weight (kg) ÷ Stature (cm) ÷ Stature (cm) x 10,000
or Weight (lb) ÷ Stature (in) ÷ Stature (in) x 703

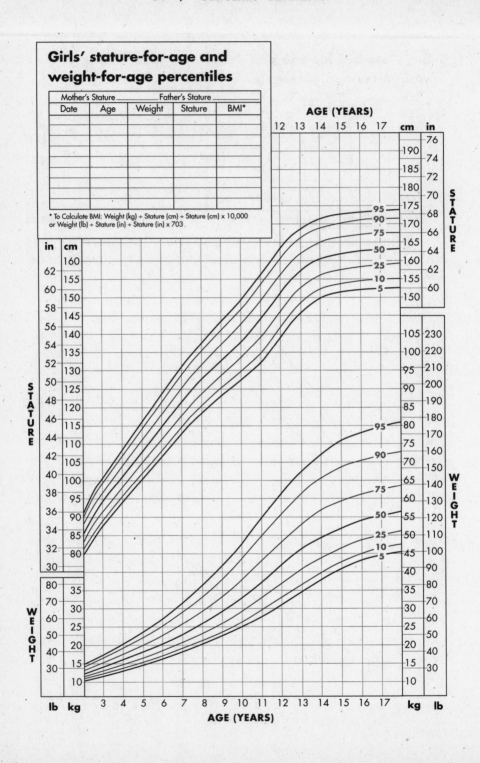

Girls' stature-for-age and weight-for-age percentiles

Mother's Stature _____ Father's Stature _____

Date	Age	Weight	Stature	BMI*

* To Calculate BMI: Weight (kg) ÷ Stature (cm) ÷ Stature (cm) x 10,000
or Weight (lb) ÷ Stature (in) ÷ Stature (in) x 703

give you is a clue, not a diagnosis. The number tells the parent and the doctor whether a child's situation merits "no concern," "some concern," or "serious concern."

The second thing to remember is that what's important about the charts is the trends they indicate with numbers plotted over *several years*, rather than any single number and percentile. A child whose BMI or weight is consistently along the 75th or 85th percentile would be less of a concern than a child whose numbers jump from the 50th to the 85th percentile over a period of several years.

That's why it's helpful to keep a copy of your child's growth chart as measured during your child's medical checkups or to plot your own at least once a year, especially if your family moves or for other reasons changes pediatricians.

PINCHING AN INCH HELPS IN READING GROWTH CHARTS, TOO

I believe the amount of body fat your hands can grab (e.g., a pinch or a handful) is a more meaningful, yet more subjective, indicator of overfatness than the child's ranking on the charts. The weight and BMI charts reflect "overweight," but not necessarily "overfat."

For example, if you have a child who plots in the 85th percentile on the weight chart, you might suspect he's overweight. But look at him. Is he a big-boned child with lots of muscle? Or are you able to grab folds of fat along his waist or under his arms? If the former, I would guess that this child need not be concerned about overfatness, especially if both his height and his weight are at the top of the chart. Rather, this child is just big. Some children can be big and lean. That is their normal and healthy body weight.

On the other hand, a child who plots in the 75th percentile for weight and BMI and the 50th for height might have more cause for concern. If you find you can pinch more than an inch at her waist or under her arms, you have some reason to be concerned.

The Dangers of a Big Middle

New insights suggest that the excess folds of fat some of us accumulate around the waist may be of greater concern than what the scale or BMI charts reflect. This abdominal fat is called "visceral fat," because what you can see around the waist is often the tip of the iceberg and is associated with a large amount of extra fat deposited beneath the surface of the abdomen. This fat is more metabolically active, which means it is released more quickly into the bloodstream—a fact that accounts for the increased risk of diabetes, high

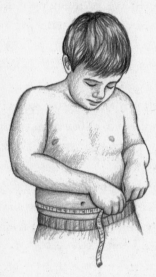

cholesterol, and cardiovascular disease among persons with excess abdominal fat. The good news is that this fat is often the first the body sheds when you begin a consistent exercise program. This is why *abdominal girth* is one of the most meaningful measurements of progress on the LEAN Kids Program. I have noticed that after a few weeks, kids on the program often report "looser pants" or "looser skirts," even without noticing a lower weight on the scale.

BALANCE THE CHART WEIGHT WITH THE CHILD'S OPTIMAL WEIGHT

In reading growth, weight, and BMI charts, another important factor to consider is the difference between the child's actual weight on the chart and his optimal weight. What I mean by "optimal weight" is what you expect the child's weight to be on the chart. As a rough rule of thumb, you would expect a child's weight percentile to be about the same as his height percentile. If your daughter is in the 50th percentile for height and the 50th percentile for weight, she is a child whose charts will indicate "no concern" to her pediatrician. (Actually, lean children often find the percentile for weight is a bit below their percentile for height. As long as the numbers are not too different, this kind of situation is not a cause for concern.)

However, suppose your ten-year-old boy plots at the 75th percentile for height and the 90th for weight. In the 75th percentile for height at age ten, you would expect him to be in the 75th percentile for weight—or about eighty pounds. But since he actually weighs one hundred pounds, he's in the 90th percentile. This child's numbers are out of balance on the charts and he could be twenty pounds, or above 20 percent, over his optimal weight. The child who weighs 20 percent more than his expected weight is considered medically obese, or at risk of becoming overfat, depending on whether or not the child has a lot of extra body fat you can see or grab. (However, if your child is strong and muscular, you should expect her to weigh more, since muscle weighs more than fat.) So in evaluating her optimal weight, you should follow a slightly different guideline than would the parent of a less muscular child. Your child's optimal weight can be as much as 10 percent higher than her height percentile.

Sometimes a child plots along the 5th percentile for weight, and parents worry that he doesn't eat enough, especially if the child has been dubbed a "picky eater." This child is either genetically petite or could be undernourished. In consultation with your doctor and a registered dietitian, you should do a *nutritional analysis*. Accurately record everything your child eats for a week, and the doctor and dietitian will compare the nutrients your child has eaten with what he needs. You may be surprised that your child is eating all he needs. In fact, the term "picky eater," while a worry for parents, is considered a benevolent term among nutritionists, since studies show that children dubbed picky eaters early on seldom grow up to be obese.

Step 2: Assess Your Child's Risk of Overfatness

Now that you understand how to read and plot growth charts, you know they are meant to be used as clues for identifying at-risk children and to follow growth trends over time; and that they are most meaningful when read not in isolation but in the context of the particular child's actual appearance and body build. With that knowledge in hand, you're ready to assess your own child's growth using the following tools.

To evaluate the status of your child's health and determine if she is overfat, you need to assess her growth according to five factors: her weight and height, her BMI, the amount of fat on her body ("pinching an inch"), her body type, and her obesity risk factors.

After you've completed these assessments, I'll show you how to use the information gathered to personalize the LEAN Kids Program for your child. Depending on your findings, you can choose a Super LEAN, Standard LEAN, or LEAN-Lite program.

1. WEIGH AND MEASURE YOUR CHILD

Weigh your child first thing in the morning, after he visits the bathroom but before his breakfast. Measure your child's height at the same time. Your child should be in bare feet and dressed only in underwear. (Although we rarely use scales in the LEAN Kids Program, when you do you should always use the same one. Even doctors' scales have individual variations that can be misleading.) This is your child's baseline starting weight and height.

(I won't ask you to weigh your child again until his next doctor visit, or about every month or two. I strongly believe that weight watching is unnecessary for a growing child, and can even set some children up for eating disorders. Keep in mind that the child's goal is not to *lose* weight but rather to maintain his current weight until his body leans out. The LEAN Kids Program is *a total health process* and not just a question of what the scale says, so you have no need to rely too much on this measurement.)

Enter the height and weight numbers in the charts on page 71 and follow the instructions on how to plot the numbers. Record the percentile rank for height and weight in the sample chart on page 71.

2. DETERMINE YOUR CHILD'S
BODY MASS INDEX (BMI)

Your child's body mass index, or BMI, is his weight (in kilograms) divided by the square root of his height in meters. That sounds complicated to compute, but it's really not. One way to do it is to refer to the growth chart you used earlier, which shows you the meters equivalent for height measurements and the kilogram equivalent for weight measurements (just look at the ruling down the sides of the chart). A calculator should be able to handle the rest.

Or if you prefer, you can use the Americanized adaptation of that formula, which is a three-step process.

1. Take your child's weight in pounds and divide it by height in inches. (For example, if she weighs sixty pounds and is fifty inches tall, the result is 1.2.)
2. Divide that result by her height in inches. (For example, divide 1.2 by 50, which will give you .024.)
3. Multiply the result by 703. (For example, .024 multiplied by 703 is 16.872.)

(The healthy range for children's BMI is lower than it is for adults. The range is age specific, so you need to refer to the chart on page 60 or 61.)

Or, if you have online access, you might want to visit www.leankids. com, where you can simply enter your child's weight and height and we'll calculate his BMI for you. Enter the BMI number in the sample graph on page 60 or 61 and in the sample chart on page 71.

Be as careful in taking your child's measurements as you can. Small errors in height or weight can lead to big errors in your child's BMI score. In fact, to be on the safe side, you might want to use all three of the methods described above. A comparison of your results will give you the most accurate score.

3. MEASURE YOUR CHILD'S FAT-COLLECTING AREAS

It's time to pinch an inch! You'll want to measure your child's waist circumference first, and be sure to do so when she is relaxed (no sucking the tummy in!). Use a soft tape measure for an accurate reading as shown on page 66.

Next, using a fat-fold caliper, you'll want to measure how much skin you can pinch into a fold at your child's fat-collecting areas. First, gently pinch a fold at his waist, where the skin is loosest. Does the fold measure more than an inch? Make a note of its exact size. Next, pinch a fold of skin under his arm and measure that.

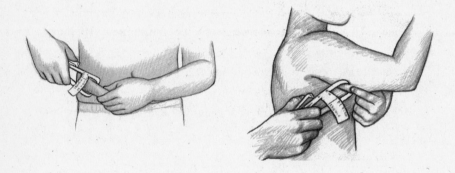

You'll want to make note of all these measurements in the chart below.

4. ASSESS YOUR CHILD'S BODY SHAPE

As we've discussed, some kids are genetically calorie burners and others are calorie storers. That means being lean will be easier for some kids than for others (although all children can achieve lean health by following the LEAN Kids Program). The question we need to answer as part of our assessment of your child's risk of overfatness is, What *is* his genetic body shape? Well, the easiest way to answer that question is to *look at your child*. While obesity is not a body shape, bigness or smallness is. So by observing your child's appearance, you should be able to evaluate whether she is a calorie burner or a calorie storer.

STARTING POINTS

Measurements	Beginning	Goal
Weight	Pounds Percentile	Pounds Percentile
Height	Inches Percentile	
BMI	Score Percentile	Score Percentile
Waist circumference	Inches	Inches
Abdominal skin fold	Inches	Inches
Triceps skin fold	Inches	Inches

Consult the Child's Doctor

After you complete the do-it-yourself charting above, you might want to take this information and your child to your pediatrician for a consultation. The doctor will also plot your child on his growth charts, evaluate the measurements, examine your child, and give you an opinion about whether or not your child is overfat and by how much. As we've discussed, some kids are just big kids, with big muscles, big bones, and a solid feel. Because these solid kids often plot proportionately higher on the weight chart than on the height chart (muscle and bone weigh more than fat tissue), you might be confused by their scores. With your doctor's help, you can avoid erroneously labeling your child "overfat."

I find it useful when assessing this issue to use a fruit and vegetables analogy for the three main body types:

- *Bananas* are tall, lean, and lanky, and tend to be calorie burners.
- *Apples* are of medium height, stocky, and have large waists.
- *Pears* tend to be slender on the top but more round in the hips and thighs.
- *Yams* are tall and thick from top to bottom, or just plain big.

Bananas find it easiest to stay lean. Apples, pears, and yams have to be more consistent about making healthy choices in order to stay lean. But they can do it. And bananas have to remember that they don't have a license to overeat. Even genetically lean children can grow up with an increased risk of cardiovascular disease and diabetes if they have unhealthy lifestyles and eating habits.

Since children equate being different with being less, it's important for children not to feel that one body type is better than the other. Just as fair-skinned kids have to be more careful about sun exposure, apples have to be more careful about what they eat. Remind your child that we all have different talents—not all great soccer players are good dancers; a math whiz shouldn't resent an artist. We should all just enjoy and nurture the talents we have. Similarly, we can all just enjoy and nurture the bodies we have.

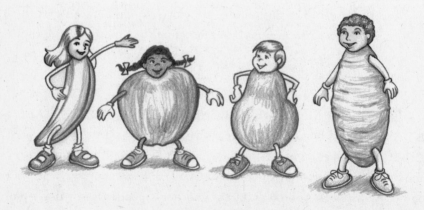

Four Kids on Four Charts

As you assess your child, it may help to consider the following four examples of children with varying degrees of leanness or fatness.

Medium Mary. Mary has a so-called medium build, as do her parents. She's a mixed fruit—a bit of a banana and a bit of an apple. She has consistently plotted around the 45th to 55th percentiles in both height and weight. With her average and balanced percentiles, Mary is in the "no concern" category.

Lean Lucy. Lucy plots high for height yet low for weight. She started out looking like an apple (being slightly above average in weight), but her banana genes clicked in as she aged and leaned out. With her weight percentile lower than her height, she is considered in the lowest-risk category for obesity.

Big Bernie. Bernie plots at the top of the class in both height and weight. He's not considered obese because his height and weight percentile *consistently plot together*. Still, since he's above the 85th percentile in weight on the growth chart, he remains at a higher risk of becoming overfat than would a child whose weight plots lower.

Fat Freddie. Freddie plots high in height, yet even higher in weight. Unlike Big Bernie, whose height and weight plot near similar percentiles, Freddie's weight just keeps climbing higher and higher until he is off the chart in weight. Even at age six, Freddie's ideal weight for his height would be less than fifty pounds, yet he weighs sixty-two pounds—or around 20 percent over his ideal weight, which is considered medically obese. Freddie is at the highest risk for becoming an obese teen and adult.

5. EVALUATE YOUR CHILD'S OBESITY RISK FACTORS

Your assessment of your child isn't complete until you assess her risk of becoming obese. Some children who don't appear fat or don't plot

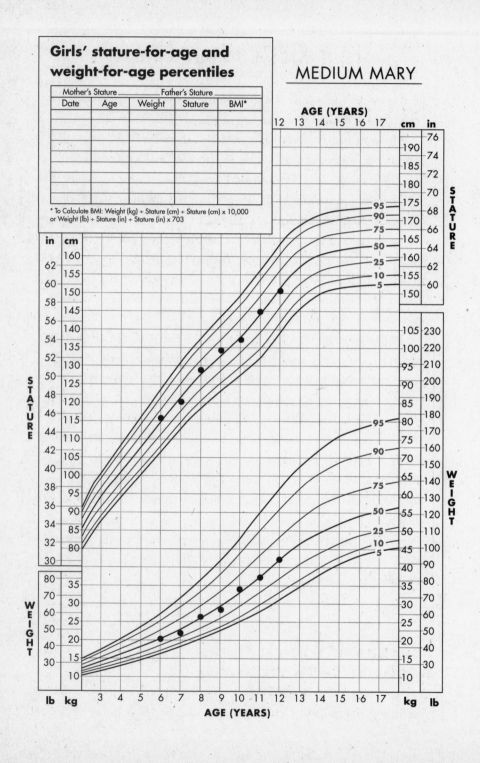

Girls' stature-for-age and weight-for-age percentiles

MEDIUM MARY

Mother's Stature _____ Father's Stature _____

Date	Age	Weight	Stature	BMI*

* To Calculate BMI: Weight (kg) ÷ Stature (cm) ÷ Stature (cm) x 10,000
or Weight (lb) ÷ Stature (in) ÷ Stature (in) x 703

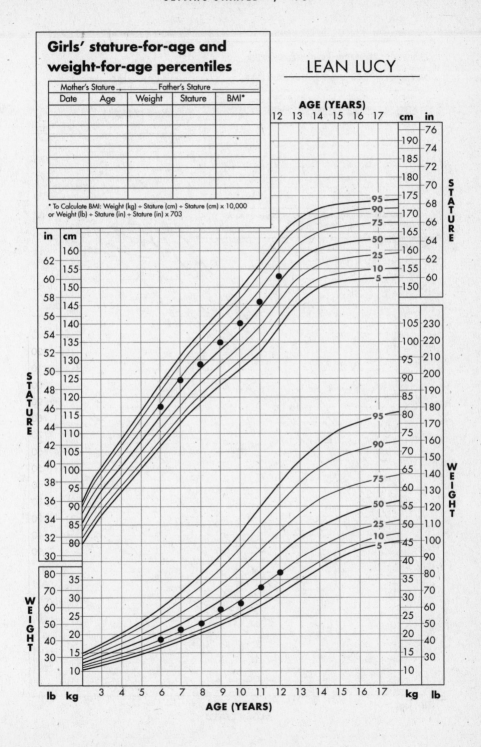

Girls' stature-for-age and weight-for-age percentiles

LEAN LUCY

Mother's Stature _____ Father's Stature _____

Date	Age	Weight	Stature	BMI*

* To Calculate BMI: Weight (kg) ÷ Stature (cm) ÷ Stature (cm) x 10,000 or Weight (lb) ÷ Stature (in) ÷ Stature (in) x 703

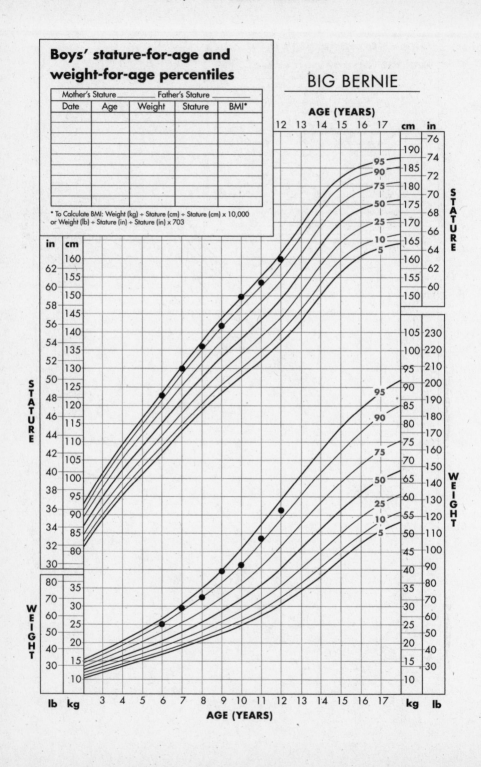

Boys' stature-for-age and weight-for-age percentiles

Mother's Stature _____ Father's Stature _____

Date	Age	Weight	Stature	BMI*

* To Calculate BMI: Weight (kg) ÷ Stature (cm) ÷ Stature (cm) x 10,000
or Weight (lb) ÷ Stature (in) ÷ Stature (in) x 703

BIG BERNIE

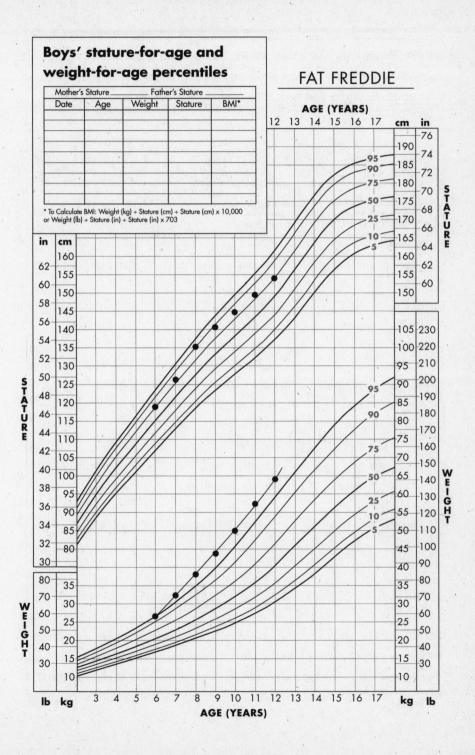

Boys' stature-for-age and weight-for-age percentiles

Mother's Stature _____ Father's Stature _____

Date	Age	Weight	Stature	BMI*

* To Calculate BMI: Weight (kg) ÷ Stature (cm) ÷ Stature (cm) x 10,000
or Weight (lb) ÷ Stature (in) ÷ Stature (in) x 703

FAT FREDDIE

significantly overweight on the charts are actually at risk for becoming overfat. You have to assess your child's risk by taking her whole picture into account. In order to do that, you can review all the assessments we have done in this chapter and match them to one of the three categories below.

RED FLAG	YELLOW FLAG	GREEN FLAG
High risk of obesity	Medium risk of obesity	Very low risk of obesity
• Parents: overweight	• Parents: one or both lean	• Parents: both lean
• Family eating habits: generally unhealthy	• Family eating habits: inconsistent, but generally healthy	• Family eating habits: consistently healthful
• Child's body type: apple; excess abdominal fat	• Child's body type: banana, slightly pear or yam	• Child's body type: banana
• Child's temperament: mostly a sitter	• Child's temperament: mover and sitter	• Child's temperament: mostly a mover
• Family tree: mostly overweight	• Family tree: mixed lean and overweight	• Family tree: mostly lean

Step 3: Assess Your Child's Physical Fitness

People use the term "fitness" to apply to everyone from Olympic-caliber athletes to super-thin models. Many parents are not sure what real fitness means, especially for their children. So I want to make it clear at the start that the LEAN Kids Program does not mean that your child needs to be-

The Risk of Being Big

Even though a big child like Big Bernie (whose height and weight are consistently in the upper percentiles of the charts) may not presently be a fat child, *a big child is always at risk for becoming fat, especially as an adult.* Big children are often not overfat, but overfed. They get away with it when they are very active, especially through adolescence. As they grow into adulthood, big children often continue to overeat but start under-exercising, which gradually leads them into obesity. Big children who are also overfat have a much higher risk of insulin resistance. Because of this risk factor, big children should always be on the LEAN Kids Program.

come a super-athlete. Rather, when I say I want children to be fit, I mean I want them to have the energy, strength, and vitality to get through their day (going to school, playing at recess, studying, and enjoying an after-school baseball game) without undue fatigue. A fit kid is one who is strong physically (meaning that she has a strong heart, lungs, and muscles) as well as strong mentally (able to handle stress and inevitable set-backs with a positive attitude).

Real fitness is not a specific body type, physique, or athletic ability. Rather, it is a state of physical well-being that helps kids live productive lives and reach their desired goals. Some children may become great athletes and require a high level of fitness to perform their specific sport. But most kids just need to have fun moving their bodies, which will help

LEAN KIDS SAY

"When I have more energy, I have more fun."
—GARRETT, AGE EIGHT

them prevent disease and accomplish their life goals. That's what fitness is all about.

In order to help you assess your child's fitness level, our fitness consultant, Sean Foy, devised seven fitness tests for you to give your child. He formulated these tests using information and data from the President's Council on Physical Fitness and Sports Norms from the Canada Fitness Award Program (Health Canada, Government of Canada). All of these evaluations are safe and easy for you to perform at home. In fact, most kids enjoy doing them!

Before you get started, be sure that before each section of the test your child has an appropriate warm-up for about ten minutes. Light stretching is a good way to start. Nonstrenuous movement is, too.

1. THE AEROBIC CAPACITY TEST: ENDURANCE WALK/RUN TEST

Purpose: To determine the strength of your child's heart and lungs by measuring its efficiency in delivering needed oxygen to working muscles.

Equipment needed: A reliable digital watch or stopwatch, available at most sporting goods stores.

Goal: To complete the designated distance in the fastest time possible by walking or running.

Instructions: Find a safe track or area that is accurately marked for the distances below. After the appropriate warm-up, on the command of "Ready, set, go," the child begins the endurance run or walk on the course you have selected. Very obese kids may prefer to walk fast rather than run.

- Ages six to seven perform a quarter-mile walk or run test.
- Ages eight to nine perform a half-mile walk or run test.
- Ages ten to eleven perform a one-mile walk or run test.

Mark your child's time in the fitness test chart on page 92.

WALK/RUN TEST

		Ages 6–7		Ages 8–9		Ages 10–12	
	Age	Distance: ¼ mile Minutes to run ¼ mile		Distance: ½ mile Minutes to run ½ mile		Distance: 1 mile Minutes to run 1 mile	
		Average	Fit	Average	Fit	Average	Fit
Boys	6	2:21	1:55			12:36	10:15
	7	2:10	1:48			11:40	9:22
	8			4:22	3:30	11:05	8:48
	9			4:14	3:30	10:30	8:31
	10					9:48	7:57
	11					9:20	7:32
	12					8:40	7:11
Girls	6	2:26	2:00			13:12	11:20
	7	2:21	1:55			12:56	10:36
	8			4:56	3:58	12:30	10:02
	9			4:50	3:53	11:52	9:30
	10					11:22	9:19
	11					11:17	9:02
	12					11:05	8:23

2. UPPER BODY STRENGTH/ENDURANCE: PULL-UP TEST

Purpose: To determine the strength and endurance of your child's upper body muscles. (Note: Your child can perform the push-up test below as an alternative to this.)

Equipment needed: A pull-up bar, which can be found at most parks or schools.

Goal: To complete as many pull-ups as possible.

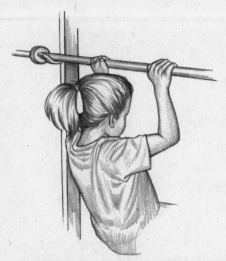

Instructions: Grasp the bar with both hands (palms facing away from the body). Hang from the bar with arms extended and without feet touching the ground. Begin the test by pulling the body up until the chin is higher than the bar. Then lower body back to the beginning hanging position. Repeat, if you can.

Record the number of completed pull-ups in the chart on page 92.

PULL-UP TEST

		Number of Pull-ups	
	Age	Average	Fit
Boys	6	1	2
	7	1	4
	8	1	5
	9	2	5
	10	2	6
	11	2	6
	12	2	7
Girls	6	1	2
	7	1	2
	8	1	2
	9	1	2
	10	1	3
	11	1	3
	12	1	2

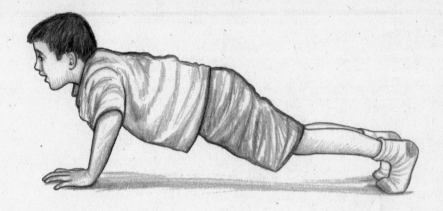

3. UPPER BODY STRENGTH/ENDURANCE: PUSH-UP TEST

Purpose: To determine the strength and endurance of your child's upper body muscles. (Note: Your child can perform the pull-up test above as an alternative to this.)

Equipment needed: A digital watch or stopwatch.

Goal: To complete as many push-ups as possible.

Instructions: This is an easily administered test for upper body strength/endurance. Your child should try to do as many consecutive push-ups as she can without stopping to rest. Instruct your child to:

- Lie on her stomach on a mat or the floor with legs together and back straight.
- Place hands pointing forward and positioned under the shoulders.
- Raise the body up by straightening the arms (keeping back and body straight).
- Lower the body until there is a 90-degree angle at her elbows. You can assist your child by placing a rolled-up towel under her chest; instruct her to touch her chest to the towel each time she lowers her body.
- Do one push-up every three seconds. Perform as many push-ups using this technique as possible without undue strain and without stopping to rest.

PUSH-UP TEST			
		Number of Push-ups	
	Age	Average	Fit
Boys	6	7	9
	7	8	14
	8	9	17
	9	12	18
	10	14	22
	11	15	27
	12	18	31
Girls	6	6	9
	7	8	14
	8	9	17
	9	12	18
	10	13	20
	11	11	19
	12	10	20

- There is no time limit. Stop the test when the child is unable to maintain proper technique or shows signs of excessive straining. Record the number of completed push-ups in the chart on page 92.

4. ABDOMINAL STRENGTH/ENDURANCE: CURL-UP TEST

Purpose: To determine the muscular strength and endurance of the abdominal (stomach) muscles. (Note: This movement is for testing purposes only and is not recommended as a regular exercise. If you would like a movement that is less strenuous on the lower back and can be used as a regular abdominal movement, see instructions for the partial curl-up test on pages 86–87.)

Equipment needed: A cushioned surface or mat, and a digital watch or stopwatch.

Goal: To complete as many curl-ups as possible in one minute. (If your child has trouble with this, see the following test as an alternative.)

Instructions: To perform this test, your child has to raise his head and shoulders off the floor and touch his elbows to the tops of his thighs. The elbows must touch the mid-thighs on the upward movement and the shoulders must touch the floor on the downward movement to qualify as a successful curl-up. Instruct your child as follows:

- On a cushioned surface or mat, lie on his back with knees bent and feet on the floor approximately twelve inches from the buttocks.
- Cross his arms, placing the hands on opposite shoulders.
- Using stomach muscles, curl upper body up until elbows touch thighs.
- Slowly lower back down until shoulders touch floor.
- To assist your child, hold his feet with your hands as you count the number of curl-ups performed in one minute. Record that number in the chart on page 92.

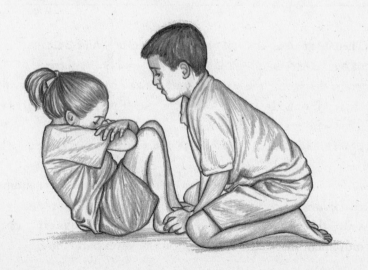

CURL-UP TEST

	Age	Number of Curl-ups	
		Average	Fit
Boys	6	22	33
	7	28	36
	8	31	40
	9	32	41
	10	35	45
	11	37	47
	12	40	50
Girls	6	23	32
	7	25	34
	8	29	38
	9	30	39
	10	30	40
	11	32	42
	12	35	45

5. ABDOMINAL STRENGTH/ENDURANCE: PARTIAL CURL-UP TEST

Purpose: To determine the strength/endurance of the abdominal (stomach) muscles. It's an alternative to the Curl-up Test and is recommended for children who are very underfit.

Equipment needed: A cushioned surface or mat and a digital watch or stopwatch.

Goal: To complete as many partial curl-ups as possible in one minute.

Instructions: Your child should perform a partial curl-up every three seconds until he cannot complete one at this pace. To begin the test, instruct your child to:

- Lie on his back on a cushioned surface or mat, with knees bent and feet on the floor approximately twelve inches from his buttocks.
- Extend his arms so that fingers rest on top of his thighs, pointing toward the knees.
- Raise his head and shoulders off the floor, sliding his hands up his legs until his fingers touch the tops of his knees. Then lower shoulders back to the floor.
- Do one partial curl-up every three seconds until he cannot maintain this pace.

PARTIAL CURL-UP TEST

		Number of Curl-ups	
	Age	Average	Fit
Boys	6	10	22
	7	13	24
	8	17	30
	9	20	35
	10	24	37
	11	26	43
	12	32	64
Girls	6	10	22
	7	13	24
	8	17	30
	9	20	33
	10	24	37
	11	27	43
	12	30	50

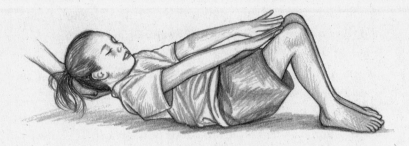

To assist your child, place your hands underneath his head so he doesn't hyperextend his neck. Record the number of partial curl-ups in the chart on page 92.

6. LEG STRENGTH/AGILITY/POWER: 30-FOOT SHUTTLE RUN TEST

Purpose: This test determines the muscular strength, agility, and power of the lower body muscles.

Equipment needed: A tape measure, masking tape or chalk, two small blocks of wood, and a stopwatch or digital watch.

Goal: To run as fast as you can four times between two lines distanced thirty feet apart.

Instructions: Select a surface that is flat and safe (ideally an indoor or outside basketball court). Using masking tape or chalk, mark one line, and then mark a second line exactly thirty feet away. Place two blocks of wood behind one line. Instruct your child to go to the opposite line. At the signal "Ready, set, go" your child should run as fast as she can to the other line, pick up one of the wooden blocks, run back to the starting line, and place the wooden block behind the starting line without throwing it. The child should then run back to retrieve the other wooden block and return to the starting line with it, placing it behind the starting line to complete the test. Instruct your child to perform this test as fast as she can without throwing the wooden blocks. Record your child's time in the chart on page 92.

30-FOOT SHUTTLE RUN TEST

		How many seconds	
	Age	Average (seconds)	Fit
Boys	6	13	12
	7	12	11
	8	12	11
	9	11	10
	10	11	10
	11	11	10
	12	10	9
Girls	6	13	12
	7	13	12
	8	12	11
	9	12	11
	10	12	10
	11	11	10
	12	11	10

7. FLEXIBILITY: V-SIT AND REACH

Purpose: To determine the flexibility of the lower back muscles and leg muscles (hamstring muscles).

Equipment needed: A ruler or measuring tape, masking tape or chalk, and a comfortable mat or surface.

Goal: To bend forward as far as possible while in a sitting position with legs in front of you.

Instructions: Select a surface that is flat and comfortable, and make a one-foot-long line on it with masking tape or chalk. Instruct your child to remove his shoes and to sit down on the floor with his legs outstretched

V-SIT AND REACH

	Age	How far they can stretch	
		Average	Fit
Boys	6	+1.0 inch	+3.5 inches
	7	+1.0	+3.5
	8	+0.5	+3.0
	9	+1.0	+3.0
	10	+1.0	+4.0
	11	+1.0	+4.0
	12	+1.0	+4.0
Girls	6	+2.5	+5.5
	7	+2.0	+5.0
	8	+2.0	+4.5
	9	+2.0	+5.5
	10	+3.0	+6.0
	11	+3.0	+6.5
	12	+3.5	+7.0

before him, placing his heels eight to twelve inches apart on the line that is marked by tape. The marked line will represent the goal to reach with his hands. It is also a reference point for you to use in measuring the distance that your child reaches.

- Instruct your child to place one hand on top of the other, both palms facing down, arms extended.
- Instruct your child to exhale, reach forward as far as he can while keeping the legs straight, and hold the reach for two seconds. Assist your child by placing your hands on top of his knees to prevent excessive bending.

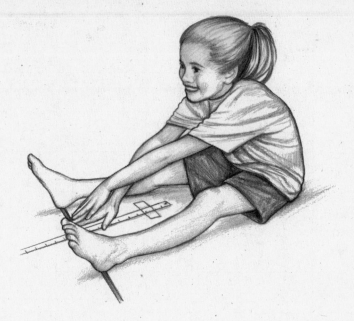

- Perform this test three times, recording the fourth attempt.
- On the fourth attempt, use the ruler to measure the distance in inches your child reaches past the line as "+" (plus) and before the line as "–" (minus). Record the distance in the chart on page 92.

EVALUATING YOUR RESULTS

In scoring each test, you noticed two columns, one indicating the "average" performance at each age and the other showing the "fit" performance. If your child falls in the "average" for all tests, he is showing a good start but may not be optimally fit. If your child scored in the "fit" range for most tests, he is showing a higher level of fitness. Regardless of where your child is right now, the goal is to use this data as a *starting point* to track progress and to motivate your child to maintain or improve upon the scores over time by being active and moving around more.

You can measure the progress your child may make in his fitness efforts by repeating these tests each month and recording your results in the chart below.

Fitness Test	Beginning Measurements	Month 1	Month 2	Month 3	Month 4	Month 5	Month 6
1. walk/run							
2. pull-up							
3. push-up							
4. curl-up (or partial curl-up)							
5. shuttle run							
6. V-sit and reach							

Step 4: Personalize the LEAN Kids Program

Now that you have a thorough assessment of your child's physical health, you can determine what level of LEAN Kids Program your child needs. While the principles of the program remain consistent in any form, it's flexible enough to meet the needs of your child. Depending on how great his risk for overfat or underfitness (and the unhappiness that goes along with them), you'll find one of the below options will be just right for him.

THE SUPER LEAN KIDS PROGRAM

The Super LEAN Kids Program involves a total commitment to the principles of the program on every level: making major *lifestyle* changes, increasing *exercise* to at least sixty minutes a day, developing a passionate *attitude* toward healthy choices, and embarking on a total makeover in *nutrition*, especially shopping and eating styles.

Your child needs the Super LEAN Kids Program if:

- She is more than 20 percent over her optimal weight on the growth chart (see how to calculate, page 69).
- His body mass index (BMI) on the charts is between the 85th and 95th percentiles or higher.
- You can grab a handful of abdominal fat folds.
- Never mind the scales, your child obviously looks overfat.
- He has red-flag risk factors as listed on page 78.
- The doctor is concerned, and she scores below average on the fitness tests.
- Everyone in your family is an apple.

THE STANDARD LEAN KIDS PROGRAM

The Standard LEAN Kids Program involves making a few lean choices each day and consistently practicing them. Most moderately overweight children can lose their excess fat by making only minor changes in their diet and moving more. For example, ten fatty potato chips a day is an extra hundred calories a day, which translates into ten pounds of extra fat a year. Lose the chips and your child will lose the excess fat. Adding twenty minutes of strenuous movement (brisk walking, playing chase, starting a sport) to his daily activities translates into burning a hundred calories of fat a day, or growing out of ten pounds of extra fat in a year. The goal on the Standard LEAN Kids Program is to make changes at a gradual pace but to be consistent about them. Keep adding new choices so that although you are changing gradually, you eventually achieve lean living in all aspects of your lifestyle, exercise, attitude, and nutrition. Base your pace on your child's temperament.

Your child needs the Standard LEAN Kids Program if:

- He is between 10 and 20 percent over his optimal weight on the growth chart and scores average on the fitness tests.
- His body mass index (BMI) on the charts is less than the 85th percentile.
- You can pinch only an inch of love handles and triceps folds.
- She has yellow-flag risk factors as listed on page 78.

- The doctor is only slightly concerned.
- Your family has a mix of different fruits for body builds.

THE LEAN-LITE KIDS PROGRAM

The LEAN-Lite Kids Program is for children who are only a few pounds overfat and who consume about 50 calories a day more than they burn. This version of the program translates into burning 50 calories more or eating 50 calories less of junk food a day so that your child can lean out over time. You can make the changes involved in adopting the LEAN Kids Program slowly, one change a day. Your child has room for some slipups, as long as you are consistently and steadily working toward changing your lifestyle, exercise, attitude, and nutritional habits. The truth is, if your child is in this group, adopting the LEAN Kids Program won't involve many changes for you or your family.

Your child needs the LEAN-Lite Program if:

- She is less than 10 percent over her ideal weight on the chart.
- You pinch less than an inch of skin on her abdomen and underarms.
- She has green-flag risk factors as listed on page 78.
- Your doctor isn't worried, and she scores in the fit category.
- Most of the people in your family are lean.

LEAN TIP

Remember, your child doesn't have to eat perfectly to eat LEAN!

Now that you've assessed your child and made baseline measurements, you are ready to use the LEAN tools to get your child healthy and fit. In the next chapter, I'll describe the first tool in the LEAN Kids Program—Lifestyle, or what I think of as healthy family habits for living lean.

6

LIFESTYLE

Live Lean

As we've discussed, the LEAN Kids Program is a total health plan that addresses the four key areas of your child's life, or what I call the four tools of the LEAN Kids Program—Lifestyle, Exercise, Attitude, and Nutrition. Let's now talk in more detail about the first LEAN tool: Lifestyle.

Lifestyle is a term usually reserved for adults and refers to the way we live. In the LEAN Kids Program, we're also referring to the daily choices we all make that contribute to a happy and healthy mind and body. In fact, in all areas of life—from personal health to relationships to career—the master success tool for adults and children is the ability to make wise choices. In the LEAN Kids Program, we think of these as healthy habits, and I want to teach you and your family to make them your own.

Top 10 Habits of a Lean Lifestyle

A healthy, lean lifestyle is made up of hundreds of little habits and choices every day. In the end, it's not so much a set of rules for living as it is behavior that stems from a thorough understanding of what makes for healthy, happy, strong children. My hope is that by the time you're done with this book, you'll have that understanding.

In order to get you there, it might help to give you a quick peek at what life might look like when you are living lean. With that in mind, I offer you the following top ten habits of a lean lifestyle—not because I want you to think of them as rules to follow, but because I think it is as good a place as any to start in helping you envision a happier, healthier life for your child. Here are our top ten habits of a lean lifestyle.

1. Grazing on nutritious foods throughout the day.
2. Making supermarket shopping a lesson in lean living.
3. Starting the day with a brainy breakfast.
4. Doing thirty to sixty minutes of physical activity daily.
5. Liking your body type.
6. Eliminating toxic or negative thoughts.
7. Spending more of the day on play time (moving) than on screen time (sitting).
8. Thinking of both eating and moving as forms of preventive medicine.
9. Getting restful sleep each night.
10. Enjoying "happy meals" with the family at least five days a week.

After reviewing these top ten habits (and especially if some of these choices are not ones you are already making), you may wonder how you are supposed to get there from here. We'll answer that question by showing you how to become your child's coach; how to talk to your child about the LEAN Program and what's involved in making a commitment to live it; and how to passionately lead the way as a role model for your child to follow toward a leaner life.

Parents As Coach

As you can see by the top ten habits of a lean lifestyle, even though the LEAN Kids Program is primarily for children it will involve the entire family—and parents must lead the way.

What if you wanted to hire a personal trainer to help you get lean? You would want your trainer to evaluate your entire lifestyle and map out

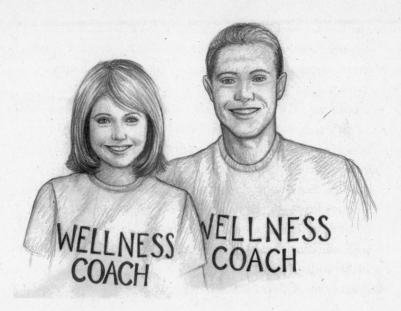

a personalized LEAN Program that met your needs. This trainer or coach would show you the most effective exercises and moves for your age and level of fitness, help you eat right to lose fat and get fit, motivate you to change your mind to change your body, and even monitor your progress and increase the program according to your progress.

We have just described your new role as your child's lean coach in the LEAN Kids Program. We want you to fully understand and appreciate the healthfulness of lean living so that you can then passionately teach what you've learned to your entire family.

COACHING TIPS

As a coach, your goal is not to control your child's eating and living habits, but rather to encourage him to have self-control—at home and away from home. To accomplish this goal, I recommend you keep the following principles in mind as you work with your child.

- *Be supportive.* Let your child know that you are proud of him even though his progress may be small or slow.
- *Be a positive role model.* Show your child you enjoy lean living yourself.

- *Don't expect perfection!* Remember, to be lean you don't have to be perfect.
- *Avoid nagging.* Try to avoid talking to your child about weight, overeating, or undereating.
- *Present the LEAN Kids Program as a wellness and lifestyle tool, not as a weight-loss program.* Remember, it's not about being thin. It's about being happy, healthy, and strong. Instead of focusing on a child's weight or fitness with statements like "to help you lose weight," "to help you get in shape," or "to help keep you from getting sick so often," try goals your child can relate to, such as "to help you run faster," "to help you make the volleyball team," and "to help you stay healthy so you don't miss as many play dates."
- *Practice the KISMIF Principle: Keep It Simple, Make It Fun!*

SHOW AND TELL

In order for your child to have the opportunity to make lean choices, the parents must be passionate about the program and agree to make lean lifestyle choices themselves. As one mom on the program said, "I realized that it wouldn't work for me to buy sodas and cupcakes for myself, yet tell my children they couldn't eat them. I'm finding I'm more a part of this program than I had thought. You *do* have to change."

Being passionate means that you care, and because you so strongly believe in the importance of health and you love your child, you are going to work against all odds to raise a lean family. Family passions are contagious. Let your children catch your passion. In fact, children love to be around passionate parents. Even if they don't agree with your chosen passions (especially when they're adolescents), they are more likely to pay more attention if you mean what you say about the LEAN Kids Program and live it yourself, rather than if you are wishy-washy about it.

PRACTICE THE WE PRINCIPLE

The We Principle is crucial to the success of the LEAN Kids Program because it shapes behavior by showing the child what you consider the normal way of living. A We attitude on your part implies a belief that

Mom Says!

Remember, while we are trying to help your child make healthy choices, the advertising media are enticing her to make unhealthy choices. Throughout the day, whenever your child is exposed to a less-than-lean message, counter with a healthier message. The TV ad says: "Junkos are good for you." Mom says: "Junkos are bad for you!" and explains why. Even if a small percentage of those daily mini-lessons sink into your child, they're worth it.

everybody lives this way. You don't have to argue for healthy choices when they are "just the way things are." Children don't like feeling different. To them, being different feels like being less. The We Principle implies that anyone who doesn't live lean is different.

Using "we" also helps you avoid sounding like a nag. Using "we" will help you convey to your child why your family believes in healthy lifestyle habits without your having to lecture about it. Try saying things like:

"This is how we eat."

"We shop the perimeter of the supermarket. We don't like the food in the middle aisles."

"We eat whole-wheat bread in our family."

"We eat fish more than hamburgers because it's better for us."

"We drink water when we're thirsty."

Add "why" to "we." You'll get a lot more mileage out of the We Principle if you also explain why your habits are healthier. School-age children want—and deserve—reasons: "We don't drink sugar-sweetened beverages in our home because these are not grow foods. They rot your teeth, upset your tummy, and can make it harder for you to fight germs."

Remember, you're competing with all the unhealthy messages from the food industry that program your children to believe that eating junk food is the norm. TV commercials, school cafeterias, and even eating at a friend's house can give your child the impression that eating white bread

Form a Lean Team

Get a group of parents together who are as motivated as you are to raise lean kids. If you and your children have friends in the same family, you might want to work with that family specifically. If the kids follow the program with friends, they'll be much more successful. You know how influential their friends are on their habits, even as very young children. If there's no one in your area with whom you can do the LEAN Kids Program, visit www.leankids.com and chat with our online community.

and sugary sodas is okay. So don't hesitate to do the "we" talk with your child as much as possible! You'll have to work pretty hard to articulate and illustrate what your family considers normal.

The We Principle is so important because it helps your child internalize the principles of living lean. In other words, if your child is continually exposed to a certain family habit, it will eventually become a natural habit in the child. The more healthy choices your child sees you make and the more healthy choices you encourage him to make throughout the day, the greater the chance that these choices will eventually become part of the child's lifestyle.

As a developmental perk, once children internalize a family habit as part of themselves, they are bothered if they are exposed to a less healthy habit. For example, a child who grew up eating mostly homemade food

LEAN KIDS SAY

"There's a kid in my class who's really fat. Her parents must not care. They let her bring marshmallows and cookies for her snack."
—LAUREN, AGE TEN

will often shun packaged food, which tastes foreign to her. A child who is taught and modeled that smoking is bad for him will be bothered by smoke and smokers. This developmental principle is known as *sensitizing* the child. On the other hand, a child who grows up in a, shall we say, polluted home isn't bothered by pollutants. This child has been *desensitized*.

SHOW YOU CARE

Children expect adults to be adults. In reading the journals kept by children on the LEAN Kids program in our pediatric practice, I was amazed to see how many children wrote that they felt parents "didn't care" when they let their children eat junk food. Because kids naturally choose food by taste and advertising, they rely on their parents to show their love by saying no to junk food when kids are unwilling to say no themselves. How willingly your child adapts to the changes in the LEAN Kids Program depends not only on how deep-seated those unhealthy habits were in the first place but also on how your child perceives your passion for raising a lean family. Counter the "But Mom!" protests with "Because Mom cares!" messages.

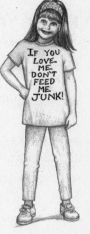

What should you say when your child protests, "Why can't I drink colas?" Your comeback could be, "Because I love you, I'm not going to let you pollute your body with that junk." Kids expect an answer like that, and it reassures them that you love them.

Choose Lean Caregivers

If your child spends a lot of time in the care of a sub, such as a baby-sitter or grandparent, you will need to instruct the sitter to support your lean lifestyle. Be clear and specific about the lean food you want your child to eat and the exercise you want your child to get.

SHAPE YOUR CHILD'S CHOICES

A parent is like a gardener. Your job as coach in the LEAN Kids Program is not to control, but rather to *shape* your children's choices. You can't control the color of the flower or the time of the year it blooms, yet you can pick the weeds and prune the plants so that they blossom more beautifully. Each day with your child is like caring for a garden. What do you water, what do you weed, and what do you prune? By *pruning* we mean weeding out unhealthy lifestyle choices that keep you from getting lean.

In addition to pruning unhealthy choices from your family, teach your children to prune for themselves. Throughout the day, whenever your child is confronted with a choice, ask, "Is this choice good or bad for your body?" Frequently offer an encouraging "Good choice!"

ADMIT YOUR MISTAKES

To be a good coach for your child on the LEAN Kids Program, you need to remember to admit your mistakes. It's essential to the success of lean living to remember that being lean doesn't mean being perfect. If you've made an unhealthy choice and suffered the consequences, let your children know: "I got so busy at work, I ate a lot of junk food, and now I feel terrible!" You might even find your child advising you to be more careful in the future, and to keep a healthy snack on hand for those overbusy days. Forgiveness breeds success.

Have the Lean Talk

As a parent and coach, you'll soon realize that translating the importance of health to your children requires a bit of creative marketing. While the ultimate goals of the LEAN Kids Program are the same for everyone, the journey will be different for each child. To begin this new lifestyle, you must first explain the meaning of lean, so your child can understand the concept of being fit and healthy. You'll need to talk openly with your child about making healthy changes. Together, you'll have to identify your child's personal challenges—the specific lifestyle choices that need changing.

The Lean Talk is obviously the place you need to start with your child. It's not only the time to introduce her to the concepts of the LEAN Kids Program, but it's also the best way to start discussing the changes in lifestyle choices that she'll need to start making. But the truth is that you can't be sure of what those changes will be until you read the rest of this book. You'll need to get all the information about lifestyle, exercise, attitude, and nutrition before you can identify the specific changes that your family needs to make. So, while I want to introduce the notion and strategy of the Lean Talk here, I need to remind you that you should not actually have this talk with your child until you've read the whole book. Once you have read the book, you will want to take the following steps in introducing your child to the LEAN Kids Program.

STEP 1: BE POSITIVE

Present the program as a get-healthy game. Don't call it a weight-loss program, because that will scare even young children. Don't let your child's first impression of the program be negative by talking about a lot of things that he can't do or eat anymore. Few children will react well if you start off by announcing, "We're going to take away all sodas and cookies" and "you can't watch so much TV." Instead, say, "We're going on a fun family bike trip" and "I found a new yummy food I want to share with you."

STEP 2: EXPLAIN LEAN

Be sure your child understands that lean does not mean "skinny" or "thin." Being thin or skinny does not always mean being healthy. In fact, a thin child may have poor eating habits, depressed immunity, and low energy, and she may not have a healthy ratio of muscle to fat.

Explain that the LEAN Kids Program is about being strong and happy. Remember that a child equates being different with being less. Because of the slim appearance of models and actors in the media, children (especially girls) can grow up thinking that being thin is cool. This child especially needs to be reminded that lean is a concept of total health, not just appearance. She'll be glad to know that the program will help her look better, but she needs to appreciate and value that it will make her stronger, too.

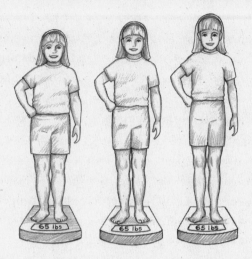

During your Lean Talk, be sure your child understands that no one body type is better than another. Naturally big kids can be as happy, healthy, and strong as naturally small kids. Lean just means achieving the right balance for your child's body. Review the discussion of body types on page 72. You might find the fruit-and-vegetable analogy I use there useful in explaining body types to your child. You want your child to like her particular body type.

Weight Loss—Not for Kids

Growing kids gain weight in muscle, bone, and other growing organs. Naturally, you want your child to lose excess fat without interfering with his normal growth. So you can't speak with children in terms of weight loss. Instead, talk about avoiding weight gain. Since the child will naturally grow in height, by setting the no-gain goal you will allow your child to simply grow into her ideal weight, or lean out.

Also, remember that there's no rush for your child to lose weight. Even more than with adults, healthful fat loss must be slow. Your child's goal should be to avoid excess weight gain and to reach a healthy weight—even if that takes years!

STEP 3: PLAY THE LIFESTYLE-CHANGE GAME

Brainstorm with your child about the specific lifestyle changes he can make that are consistent with the LEAN Kids Program. If your child helps you come up with these ideas, he'll be more enthusiastic about trying them.

Of course, the changes you come up with will depend on your personal lifestyle—and you'll get more ideas about what you may need to change as you read through the rest of this book. So wait until you're finished to take this step with your child. But for now, just to give you an idea of how to handle the Lean Talk, here are some changes that children on the LEAN Kids Program in my pediatric practice have made.

- If your child hates getting up early on school mornings and is too rushed to eat a nutritional breakfast, try moving her bedtime up by fifteen minutes and setting her alarm clock for fifteen minutes earlier each morning. She'll be surprised by how much difference such a small adjustment can make.
- If your child still complains that she doesn't have enough time for a big breakfast, make her a nutritional smoothie such as Schoolade (see page 206). If you get it ready for her, she can be out the door on time and still get the benefits of a balanced, brainy breakfast.
- If he is addicted to computer games after school, challenge him to spend no more of his day on screen time than he does on moving time. Explain that "moving" includes walking, climbing stairs, playing at recess—a lot of things he already does as part of his day. That will make the concept of "screen time equals moving time" less scary. But also point out that if he wants to play a *lot* of Game Boy, he'll have to add more moving time to his day as well. (In the exercise chapter, you'll get specific ideas about how to help him do this.)
- If your child has been exercising her mind all day at school but is not moving her body, challenge her to some "home play" before she does her homework. Moving the body helps pump more blood to the brain and actually gets the whole central nervous system in the right physiologic mood to do homework more

efficiently. (Again, the chapter on exercise will give you specific ideas about how to do this.)

- If your child is reluctant to try a sport, suggest that you learn it together. One mother I know didn't learn how to ice skate until she took lessons with her six-year-old son. The best part for him was that he learned faster than she did and ended up the better skater. There's no better confidence booster for a child than beating Mom around the rink!

- Show your child a list of healthy foods (see page 167) and ask him to pick three foods on it that he likes. Then be sure to have those foods readily and easily available to him for snacking. I've always believed that 90 percent of the reason kids eat junk food is because it's easy—you just grab the bag, rip it open, and eat. Leave a bowl of fruit on the kitchen counter. If you make eating healthful foods just as easy, you might find that your child happily eats more of them.

- If healthful foods are unfamiliar to your child, make a game out of trying one new food a week. Pick foods from the recommended list on page 167, and try to prepare them in ways you think your child will enjoy. For instance, if your child's favorite food is pasta with sauce, trying using a whole-wheat pasta with the same sauce. He'll probably like it just as much!

- One patient of mine was a ten-year-old girl who really hated her pear-shaped body type. No matter how much her mother told her how beautiful she was, she was very negative about her appearance. Then her mom had the idea of making a collage of photographs from magazines showing pear-shaped models. (The truth is, the curvaceous lines of the female pear body type are starting to be pretty popular again!) Her daughter loved the art project and was surprised by how many beautiful women had the same body type she did. She's loved her natural look ever since.

These are just some ideas that have worked for my patients, but I hope they give you ideas about how you can have fun working with your child to make the lifestyle changes involved in lean living.

STEP 4: EMPHASIZE WISE CHOICES

The ability to make wise choices is one of the most important success tools in life, and kids like choices. Having a choice gives a child a sense of control of her own body and her own destiny. Choices make him feel like a valuable participant rather than a puppet. Your children are more likely to follow the program if they feel they have choices than they are if you just tell them what to do.

When you present the LEAN Kids Program to your children, explain it as a way for them to make smart choices. And instead of telling your child what to do, offer as many choices as you can. For example, avoid saying, "Don't eat that Twinkie. Choose an apple for a snack." Instead, ask, "At school, did you choose an apple or a Twinkie for your snack?" If your child makes an unhealthy choice (which will happen!), don't scold her or tell her which choice she should have made. Instead, ask, "Is that the healthiest choice you could make?" You might even ask her, "What nutritional benefits does a Twinkie give you? What does an apple give you? Which is better?" Helping kids to weigh the pros and cons of making lifestyle choices will help them learn to make healthy choices for the rest of their lives.

A Change a Day Keeps the Doctor Away

Making small changes can add up to big health benefits, especially for kids. Why? Because kids naturally use around 25 percent of their calories to grow, so they are naturally fat-burning machines. If your child is less than enthusiastic about the LEAN Kids Program, ease into it by asking him to make just one lean change each day. Within a month you'll have a lean home and a leaner child. Even though the child may continue not to live and eat lean when away from home, he'll benefit from the changes you've made in your family's lifestyle.

STEP 5: PERSONALIZE YOUR CHILD'S LEAN CHOICES

The lifestyle changes necessary can seem overwhelming at first to both you and your child—especially if you haven't been making many lean choices in the past. The best way to avoid this feeling is to focus on your child. At this point in the Lean Talk, you and your child should identify the personal habits that need changing. Brainstorm lifestyle changes that will help him make those changes.

Remind your child (and yourself) that despite the tons of advice in this book, the LEAN Kids Program boils down to four simple concepts:

1. *Live Lean:* Make healthy choices a habit.
2. *Move Lean:* Move your body for 30 to 60 minutes each day.
3. *Think Lean:* Be positive with yourself and others.
4. *Eat Lean:* Eat healthfully.

Even if your child makes only one change in each category, she is on the way to becoming lean. She can achieve success quite easily by adding personal goals, one at a time, to these basic program principles.

There are a couple of different strategies for identifying your child's personal needs. You might, for instance, start by listing the habits your child currently has that are causing him problems. (You'll have a better idea of what should go on this list after you've reviewed the whole book. Remember, you should finish the book before embarking on this Lean Talk with your child.)

Make a chart and put the list of unhealthy habits that you and your child come up with on the left-hand side. Then, on the right-hand side, brainstorm new choices your child can make to change that unhealthy habit into a healthy one.

Here's an example of one of my patients' Personal Goal charts.

UNHEALTHY CHOICE	HEALTHY CHOICE
Lifestyle: Sits a lot in front of TV and computer	I follow the "moving equals sitting" rule at home.
Exercise: Not involved in any after-school sport	I try at least three after-school activities. My parents let me choose what sport to do as long as I stick with it for at least one season.
Attitude: Complains a lot about bad things that happen during the day	I enjoy playing a game at dinner where each family member has to mention three good things that happened during the day.
Nutrition: Eats a lot of sugared snacks	I eat fresh fruit Mom or Dad makes available to me instead of snacking on junk food.

STEP 6: TAP INTO YOUR CHILD'S PERSONAL PASSIONS

To identify your child's personal goals on the LEAN Kids Program, find out what she most wants to achieve. Even though your child may want to look thinner and wear fashionable clothes, children seldom get lean for reasons of body image alone. In addition, unlike adults, children are not motivated by the idea of living longer. Kids are totally performance oriented. In order to get your child to make healthy changes, you need to find out your child's *internal motivator.*

Every child has a special something he can do well and cares most about. Whatever skill, talent, or interest your child may have, recognize that it can work as a powerful motivator for change.

For example, here is a list of personal goals some of my patients had when they started the LEAN Kids Program in my practice. These are the things the kids themselves said they wanted to accomplish by joining the program:

- "I want to run faster so I can play better on the soccer team."
- "I'm not doing as well in math this year because it's at the end of the day now, and I'm always too tired to pay attention."
- "I don't want to be sick and miss school so often. I miss my friends."
- "I don't want my jeans to feel so tight on my tummy."

Whatever your child's personal goal in his young life, take it and go with it. Show your children how making lean choices can help them reach that goal. They'll be highly motivated, and the success they achieve will help you to expand their commitment to the LEAN Kids Program. I call this the "carry over" effect. Succeeding in one area will boost your child's self-confidence, which will empower her and inspire her to believe that she can succeed in other areas as well. Before long, you'll find your child eager to make more and more of the LEAN Kids Program her way of life.

Wow Your Child!

How much is ten pounds of body fat? Answer: one basketball full. Imagine your child having to lug around a basketball full of excess fat. I call this a "wow" lesson. As you're teaching your child how to live lean, paint word pictures to help him understand what you're talking about. "Wow" lessons sink in.

STEP 7: MOTIVATE YOUR CHILD

By the time kids are school-age (and especially if your child has a weight and fitness problem), unhealthy habits are probably already an ingrained lifestyle. When that's the case, you might have trouble motivating your child to make the changes required to start living lean. In my experience, once a child experiences some of the benefits of the LEAN Kids Program, she will have all the motivation she needs to embrace more. But it can be hard to get some children started. If the personal goal chart above doesn't work and tapping into your child's personal passion doesn't help, here are some backup strategies for getting your child started on a lean lifestyle.

Use reverse psychology. Depending on your child's personality, you might want to try a bit of reverse psychology. When you serve a new food at dinner, don't offer him any. Don't say it's not allowed; just don't discuss it. Serve yourself and be obvious about your enjoyment. Wait until he asks for a bite off your plate. It's more likely he'll admit he likes the food if he does. (This tactic works best if, while you are trying a new food, you serve your child a familiar food he eats but is not particularly fond of.)

Get serious about healthy foods. If your child turns up his nose to every food on the recommended lists in the nutrition chapter, you might have to try tougher tactics. If you don't buy junk food and stock it in your pantry, your child won't get junk food at home. Stop buying junk foods. Just get them out of your house. There should be nothing to eat in your pantry but healthy foods. Serve your child only the lean foods you eat. Serve them in *small* portions. If she refuses to eat them, or eats only a small amount, don't scold her. But also don't prepare her alternative (less healthy) meals. Eventually, she will get hungry enough to try what you are serving her.

The hunger drive is so strong that children offered food *will not go hungry.* Reassure her that you love her and that's why you want to see her eat food that will help her grow. Once the healthy foods you serve become more familiar to her, she'll start to like them. Studies show that children will eventually accept a food that they originally rejected; yet they may need to be exposed to that new food twenty times. Don't give up!

Use the three-bite rule. If the natural, whole foods in the LEAN Kids Program are completely new for your family, you'll face the extra hurdle of just getting your children to try them. Linda Chan, the registered dietitian who held classes on lean eating in our pediatric practice, advocates the three-bite rule. She tells the kids she works with, "Take three bites, and you'll discover how good it is. If you don't like it, you don't have to eat any more, and we'll try it again when you're a bit older."

Your own reactions to the new foods on your family dinner table are important, too. Avoid counterproductive statements like "You probably won't like it." Never frown or say "This looks weird" when you see a new or different food—both are guaranteed turnoffs. Instead, try a more positive approach. Show enthusiasm when you try a new food. You might find it's contagious.

Take Lean Action

The first step in starting a lean lifestyle is to become your child's coach and to have the Lean Talk with him. The next step is beginning lean living by making real changes in your family's choices and habits. While later chapters will discuss changes you need to make in your exercise, attitude, and nutritional habits, let's focus now specifically on some lifestyle changes you can make.

LEAN OUT YOUR REFRIGERATOR AND PANTRY

Take a careful inventory of your refrigerator and pantry. Compare it to the lists of healthy foods in the nutrition chapter. How many unhealthy foods do you have in your house? Make a new kind of shopping list— one that lists all the foods recommended in this book for you to choose from when you shop (see chapter 9). You might want to go to a bookstore or library and explore lean cookbooks. Find some recipes that will create more healthful meals for your family, and start stocking your house with foods for lean living.

At the same time, make a commitment to purging unhealthful foods from your house. If you and your family have been eating primarily junk and packaged foods until now, you'll need to make these changes gradually. I recommend replacing one junk-food staple with a healthful staple each week. First, buy whole-wheat bread instead of white bread. Next week, buy and clean carrots for your kids to snack on and stop buying packaged chips. You'll get more ideas about what to do from the nutrition chapter. Just make a list of the good foods and take it one step at a time.

TAKE YOUR CHILD SHOPPING

Use the supermarket as a giant nutritional classroom. There are lean lessons—good and bad—in every aisle. To raise a lean shopper, try the following suggestions:

Shop the perimeter. That's where most of the lean foods (or whole foods) are, such as fruits, vegetables, dairy, fish, and meats. Show your child that most of the food in the center aisles (the "fat" of the store) comes in cans, bottles, boxes, and bags. That means someone else has mixed foods together and put them in a container (a package). Usually that means they've taken nutritious ingredients out and added things we don't need or want.

Play label games. Teach your child how to read ingredient labels. Explain that if sugar (or corn syrup) is one of the first four ingredients, the food isn't good for us. Explain how to check for good words (like "whole grain") and bad words (like "hydrogenated" or any chemical with a number sign, like "red #40"). Explain that strange words that are hard to read are usually chemical names and indicate that the food isn't good for us.

Play color games. Let children select their own veggies. "Go pick out two reds, three greens, two yellows." Give them more points for the deep, rich colors they find on vegetables than for the pale, see-through lettuce.

Where's the sugar? This is a shopping game you can play with cereals. Most of the kids doing the LEAN Kids Program with our pediatric practice just love it. Start by showing your children the nutrition facts box on a packaged cereal. Show them where it says "carbohydrate," and explain that the grams given are for all the different kinds of carbs in each serving, both healthy and unhealthy. Then show them the sugars line, which is supposed to report how much sweetener has been added by the manufacturer. But the real story is between the lines. There are two important numbers that give you a clue as to whether the product is nutritious or in the junk category. The wider the difference between the total carbohydrates and the sugar numbers on the label, the more nutritious are the carbs in the food.

For instance, on the label for a healthy cereal, you'll see something like 24 grams of carbohydrates and 6 grams of sugar. A less nutritious cereal contains 28 grams of total carbohydrates and 15 grams of sweeteners. That means over 50 percent of the total carbs are just plain sugar.

Teach your kids to look for a ratio of 3 grams of total carbs for each 1 gram of sugar on the label if they want to consider the packaged food good for them. (These numbers work only when you're looking at cereals; they don't apply to other packaged foods.)

Read the fine print. Teach your child to ignore the hyped words on the front of packaged foods. Food manufacturers love to splash words like "natural," "pure," and "enriched" on their boxes because they know that consumers don't realize that these words have no legal meaning. They love to declare a product "low fat," without confessing that it is also "high sugar." Tell your child to ignore all this fancy packaging, and pay attention only to the ingredient list and nutritional fact box when selecting packaged foods.

Teach comparison shopping. Children like challenges. Ask your child to compare a box of nutritious cereal with a box of junk cereal. Notice that the healthy cereal contains more protein, fiber, and healthy carbs in fewer calories, so it is more "nutrient dense" than the junk cereal. Help her identify these differences in the labels. Compare two different containers of yogurt (which should be a healthy food but often isn't). Ask your child to compare a plain yogurt (you could add your own fresh fruit) with a sweetened one. The unsweetened yogurt contains more protein and calcium and fewer calories, so it is more "nutrient dense" than the sweetened yogurt. Help him identify these differences in the labels.

Let kids write the list. Once you've taken your children shopping the lean way a few times, I encourage you to let them help plan your shopping list. Offer them lots of healthy suggestions, but let them pick the breakfasts, lunches, snacks, and even some of the dinners you'll eat in the coming week. It will help them practice their lean lessons. And children are much more likely to actually eat the foods they choose themselves.

"Air Bread"

Next time you and your child are in a supermarket, go to the bread rack. Place a loaf of white bread in one of your child's hands and a loaf of whole-grain bread in the other hand. Ask your child, "What difference do you feel?" Most children will notice that the whole-grain loaf is heavier. "That's because it has a lot more real food in it than the white bread, which is full of a lot of air," you explain.

EAT LEAN WHILE EATING OUT

Eating lean at a restaurant requires some effort on your part. Look at it from the restaurant owner's point of view. The bottom line is profit. Patrons choose food primarily for taste, so the owner is motivated to serve high-fat, high-sugar, and salty meals made with the least expensive ingredients, so that he can serve big portions that are perceived as a big value. All that spells trouble for you and your kids.

Fast-food restaurants might seem like the obvious problem to you, but the truth is that even gourmet restaurants aren't always safe. I heard about a chef at a top New York eatery who routinely ladled a spoonful of melted butter on top of every entrée that left the kitchen. He said it guaranteed that customers would "just love it."

So, what is a lean eater to do? Try these tips:

Fill up on salad first. Choose a restaurant that has a salad bar or serves salad before the main entrée. Dark green lettuce and fresh vegetables are full of fiber and are filling, which sets you up to avoid overeating. Just be sure to go easy on the salad dressing.

Beware of buffets. Kids love buffets because of their enormous quantities and the olfactory delights that tempt the senses. And that's just what makes them fattening. The child walks around the table, and the aroma of all those foods will tempt her so much that she's likely to forget the LEAN Kids Program. If there's no avoiding a buffet, try to use the experience to present an important lean lesson. As you walk around the table of temptations, ask your children to show you the healthy foods for their plate. Also ask them to show you the unhealthy foods they should avoid.

Forget kids' menus. It's a sad fact that kids' menus are junkier than adult menus. Restaurant owners assume that kids don't have a taste for nutritious foods and parents are unwilling to insist that they make healthy choices. So let your child selectively order off the adult menu. Ask for a smaller portion or split an adult portion between two children. Make it clear to the restaurant that you don't appreciate the message that children are second-class eaters.

LEAN KIDS SAY

"They never have salads on kids' menus. That's why
I always order off the adult menu, because the foods taste better
and are a lot healthier for you. It's so sad how kids have
such bad food on kids' menus."
—JACOB, AGE NINE

Use the "instead of" approach. When you're reading a fast-food menu with your kids, use the opportunity to teach another lean lesson I call the "instead of" approach. This tactic gives them more control over their food choices. Suggest to your children, "Instead of French fries, try a side order of fresh fruit." Or "Instead of a cola, try the 100 percent juice." Even at dessert time, you can suggest, "Instead of ice cream, try frozen yogurt."

Grill the waiter. No, not over an open flame, but about the quality of the food. Don't be embarrassed to ask about the ingredients used in a dish. Ask for the sauce on the side. At fast-food restaurants, if you're uncertain of the nutritional content of a particular food, such as a bun or a salad dressing, ask for a printed nutritional breakdown. Most popular fast-food chains have these.

Order healthy choices. Study the menu for lean meats that are broiled or grilled, and avoid anything fried. Look for sauces that are tomato-based rather than cream- or butter-based. Ask for whole-grain bread and olive oil instead of white bread and butter. Be prepared for the occasional "aw, Mom" statement of embarrassment from your child. You have the opportunity here to teach your child an important lean lesson in life: The more often restaurant patrons ask for nutritious foods, the more they're likely to get them. You not only get what you pay for, you get what you ask for.

Keep a list of lean restaurants. Keep a record of the restaurants you find in your area that will accommodate your lean requests. "Kid-friendly" should not mean the restaurants with entertainment, video games, and kids' junk menus. Your kid-friendly restaurants should be the ones that are friendly to your family's lean way of eating. And nothing will get the message to restaurateurs about how important lean

Shun Value Meals

Fast-food chains like to brag about their "value meals," but the value is all to them in profits and not to you in nutrition. Kids don't get fat on burgers alone. They get fat on the fries and sugary sodas that come along as part of most kids' meals. To fatten their profits, fast-food chains combine their low-profit items (like burgers and fish) with high-profit servings of French fries and soda. Don't be tempted to buy jumbo drinks and value packs for your child just because it looks as if you get more for your money. In terms of nutrition, your child is getting less. In terms of her waistline, she's getting more than she needs.

eating is to customers than spending your dollars at the places that serve healthful foods.

Make a stand. Parents, you are at the top of the food chain when it comes to restaurant food. If you order it, they will serve it. Don't blame fast-food chains for the fattening of American kids. After all, McDonald's tried a McLean line. It flopped because parents didn't order it. Spend your dollars where the food is healthy, and before long we'll all have more lean restaurants to eat in.

STAY LEAN WHILE ON VACATION

Vacations are not as much of a risk to lean living as you might fear. A fact of family vacations is that even though you eat more, you also tend to move more. Chances are that because you will be burning more calories through swimming, playing games, dancing, and other activities, the excess food you eat may not translate into extra fat. However, here are some pre-vacation precautions you and your family can take.

Pre-lose. Knowing that overeating and indulging is part of a vacation, spend a couple of weeks preparing for a lapse by dropping a couple of pounds. This is especially important when you are planning nonactive vacations. It's easy to lean off a pound or two during the two weeks before your vacation. Then you don't need to worry about gaining a little while you're away. And not worrying so much is the whole point of a vacation, isn't it?

Continue to make wise food choices. Chances are that the lean habits you have learned will prompt you to eat wisely on vacation, too. Just be sure you and your children don't take a vacation from your good sense. If you abandon your lean lifestyle and gobble down French fries and cream pies for a week, you will be setting yourself up for problems when you get home. But don't worry too much about slipping up like this. The fact is that if you've been living lean at home for any length of time before you go on vacation, you won't *want* those high-fat, high-sugar foods while you're away any more than you do when you're at home.

LOBBY FOR A LEAN SCHOOL

Schools, like homes, are supposed to give children tools to succeed in life. Yet most schools get a failing grade when it comes to teaching children about health. Budget pressures have led many schools to cancel or shorten their physical education programs and after-school sports programs. Few schools still offer regular health classes. And schools give kids the fattening message that the four food groups are Burger King, Pizza Hut, McDonald's, and KFC.

Many parents are quick to voice their opinion when the school doesn't meet the academic standards they expect for their children. There are school programs for sexually transmitted diseases (STDs) and drug abuse. Yet the disease consequences of obesity pose greater social and health problems than poor reading scores, drugs, or STDs.

Parents are at the top of the food chain. Want to give your child's school a passing grade for health? Here are some ways you can help get your child's school lean:

Get involved. Join the PTA and form a lean team of other parents to improve your school's health habits. You'll need to lobby for a healthier cafeteria, because these changes will cost money. You should also encourage the PTA to look at the school's physical education program and make suggestions for improving it. The bottom line is that to get a voice in how your child's school is run, you have to take the time and effort to join the PTA.

Get fast-food chains out of your school. Fast-food chains are literally bribing schools for access to their students' dollars for lunchtime meals. Your first job on the PTA should be to organize the parent body to make it clear to the school administration that your children's health is not for sale!

Get lean food into the vending machines. Insist on 100 percent juices and bottled water instead of sugary, high-caffeine sodas in the school vending machines. In a study of low-income-population schools, replacing vending machines containing sweetened beverages with water coolers resulted in decreased obesity. Remember, besides learning eating habits in school, children also learn drinking habits.

LEAN KIDS SAY

"The food kids bring in their lunch boxes really isn't much better than the food the cafeteria has. For example, one kid brought a hot dog in his lunch box for lunch. For a drink he had Coke. Another time he had a cold bacon burger and Coke. He did not have any fruits or vegetables. This particular kid has a major weight problem. I am sad for him, because his mom doesn't pay attention to what he eats."

—LAUREN, AGE TEN

Making healthy lifestyle changes and developing healthy habits is essential for your LEAN Kids Program. Now that you have learned how to act as your child's coach, how to get her started on the LEAN Kids Program with a Lean Talk, and how to make some tangible changes in your family's choices and habits to start living lean, it's time to turn to the next tool in the LEAN Kids Program: Exercise.

7

EXERCISE

Move Lean

Move! That's one of the magic words of the LEAN Kids Program. Just as you coached your child in how to make healthy lifestyle changes, you can help him discover that *the more you move, the better you'll feel.* As you have learned, the two main reasons that children become overfat, under-fit, and unhappy is that they are eating too much junk food and moving too little.

In the exercise part of the LEAN Kids Program, we'll show you how to help your child—and the entire family—enjoy the feel-good and lean benefits of getting those little—and big—bodies moving. We will show you how to turn your child off of the PlayStation and on to the play-ground!

Before You Start

What images come to your (and your child's) mind when you hear the word "exercise"? Having a coach yell at you to run faster? Jogging mile after mile while training for a competition? Doing push-ups until your muscles scream in pain? For many, the thought of exercise evokes feel-ings of inadequacy. This is especially true for children, who are often forced into physical activities they don't like. (*You* get to choose what you do—and wear—at your gym. In gym class, your child doesn't!)

All this negative baggage about exercise really isn't necessary. There are ways to make moving a joyful part of your life. That's what I want to show you in this chapter. The LEAN Kids PLAY Program is the key to the beginning of a more active life for your child, but before we get started, there are a few things you should know that will help put the whole idea of exercise in a more positive light.

PLAY IT SAFE!

The first step to beginning any program of physical activity is to make sure you're ready for it. While the fitness assessment in chapter 5 will give you a good idea of where your child falls on the fitness chart, I recommend that you consult your child's healthcare provider prior to beginning this or any other fitness program, especially if your child is under medical supervision for a special condition, such as frequent chest pains, high blood pressure, obesity, diabetes, liver or kidney disease, or muscle, joint, or bone problems that might be aggravated by exercise. If your child is currently under a physician's care for any disease or illness, physician clearance as well as specific guidance and recommendations are highly recommended. The same holds true for you!

THE NO PAIN, NO GAIN MYTH

Many parents and children alike are still suffering from the misunderstanding that exercise needs to be painful, boring, and time-consuming to work. Remember the old adage, "No pain, no gain"?

Well, that was yesterday's thinking. New evidence has shown that low to moderate physical activities (climbing stairs, recreational sports, or even household activities such as gardening) performed throughout a busy day can have significant long-term health benefits. In fact, the bottom line is that exercise can be fun and still build a stronger and smarter body.

REMEMBER WHAT EXERCISE CAN DO FOR YOU AND YOUR CHILD

If you're still feeling a little reluctant to embark on an exercise program with your child, let me try to motivate you by reminding you of the benefits such a change has to offer you and your family.

Exercise increases a positive attitude. As soon as you and your child start moving more, you'll feel better about yourselves. We know that kids who move their bodies more experience higher self-esteem and a better feeling of general well-being than do kids who are couch potatoes.

Exercise is a remedy for unhappiness. Both aerobic exercise (brisk walking and running, for example) and strength training reduce depression. Research has also documented the fact that regular exercise releases "good feeling" hormones like endorphins. Fifteen to thirty minutes of exercise, every other day, can help depressed people enjoy frequent positive mood swings within two to three weeks.

Exercise enhances life skills. Children who participate in interscholastic sports are less likely to smoke or use drugs and are more likely to stay in school, maintain good conduct, and reach high academic achievement. Active sports and physical-activity programs also have been shown to introduce kids to much-needed life skills, such as effective communication, leadership, teamwork, sportsmanship, conflict resolution, and goal setting. Research also indicates that a lack of recreational activity may contribute to making kids more susceptible to negative influences such as drugs, gangs, or violence. (For more health benefits of exercise see page 245.)

Convinced? Then let's get started!

Move More, Think Better!

A Canadian study compared kids who moved their bodies regularly (performing vigorous activity five times per week) with kids who did not move regularly (performing less than two hours of activity per week). Not only did the active children improve their health and fitness by increasing their muscular strength and cardiovascular endurance, but they also improved their academic performance in languages, math, and sciences. Like Grandma said, "A sound body is a sound mind."

The LEAN Kids PLAY Program

The LEAN Kids PLAY Program has a unique approach to fitness for the entire family. We've coined the term PLAY for referring to exercise or movement because it is an acronym for the following four elements:

Physical activity,

Lengthening movements,

Active sports (aerobic activities), and

Youthful, kidlike strength movements

These are the four types of activities that make up the LEAN Kids PLAY program. Within each group of activities, we will provide you with specific suggestions for things your child can do to start moving. The idea is that you and your child can try a wide variety of activities and choose to practice regularly the ones you like best. Your goal is to devise a personalized PLAY program that is both fun and healthy. Let's get started!

PHYSICAL ACTIVITY

The first of the four elements in our program include play movements—in other words, moving just for the fun of it. These aren't formal physical exercises. It's just an acknowledgment that the ordinary moving we do throughout the day has health benefits, too. These physical activities include any bodily movements that cause the muscles to move and expend energy, such as taking the stairs instead of the elevator, walking to and from school, walking the dog, or going for a leisurely family stroll.

LEAN KIDS SAY

"But Dad, shopping is a sport! You have to walk a lot around the mall and sometimes run fast to get to the store before it closes."

—LAUREN, AGE TEN

The benefit of play movements. This kind of moving has the same benefits as more formal physical exercise. It can help with weight control, prevent heart disease, reduce cholesterol levels and the risk of diabetes, strengthen bones, lower the risk of certain cancers, and help to manage stress.

Frequency of activity. Encourage your child to engage in moving and play activities for thirty to sixty minutes throughout the day.

Choose from the PLAY activity list. Here's a list of daily activities you and your child can incorporate into your day for as much as an hour of play movement. You're probably doing a lot of this already! But if you don't move for at least an hour a day, you might want to try some of these suggestions to move more:

- Walk with your family in your neighborhood
- Have a pillow fight with the kids
- Throw a Frisbee
- Toss a softball or baseball
- Play a basketball game
- Have a blast with some hula hoops
- Flip on music and dance
- Go for a family hike in the country
- Take the stairs
- Jump rope with your kids
- Invite your child to participate in household chores with you
- Teach your child to roller-skate
- Play leapfrog, tag, or hide-and-seek
- Ride a bike to and from school
- Garden together

LENGTHENING MOVEMENTS

Now that you've been introduced to the "P" in the PLAY Program, let's talk about "L," which stands for lengthening moves. Lengthening movements include slow, relaxed, and focused *stretches* that take a muscle to a point of mild tension and hold the stretch (without bouncing) for a period of fifteen to thirty seconds. (See exercises, page 127.)

The benefit of lengthening movements. To understand how important lengthening movements are, think of your child's muscles as rubber bands. (In fact, when presenting to your child the importance of keeping muscles flexible, it is a good idea to use a rubber band as a visual aid.) Grasp the band in your hands and slowly pull it. Notice how the rubber band gets tighter. Our muscles are the same. As muscles stretch, they also tighten. At some point the rubber band will snap. Likewise, muscle injuries can increase dramatically when muscles are tight and limited in flexibility. Teaching children lengthening movements will help prevent injury now as well as in the future. Lengthening movements improve muscle flexibility, strengthen tendons and ligaments, increase joint mobility, improve body posture and body symmetry, decrease lower back pain, delay muscle fatigue, minimize muscular soreness after activity, decrease stress, and increase blood circulation.

Frequency of activity. Encourage your child to perform three to eight lengthening movements, three to five days a week.

Prepare the muscles. Always warm up with at least five minutes of light exercise, such as jogging in place, before stretching. Warm muscles become more flexible and less prone to injury.

Choose your moves. You and your child should choose three to eight daily stretches from the list below. Each of the exercises is performed the same way: Don't bounce, hold for fifteen seconds, and repeat each stretch two times. Pick as few as three stretches to start with. Never drop any—just add new stretches to the ones you already do. Try to do them three to five times a week. Always do them at least two times a week. Stretching is a use-it-or-lose-it game.

ACTIVE SPORTS AND AEROBIC ACTIVITIES

Your children are now working their way up the PLAY stairs. The "P" and "L" steps help get their muscles (and minds) into the *habit* of moving. These two steps are necessary for healthy and strong muscles, but they don't make them a whole lot stronger. The more intense movements of the "A" and "Y" steps not only burn fat but also build strength.

For years, teachers and coaches alike have tried to get kids in shape by prescribing long, grueling, aerobic conditioning programs that were

Lengthening Exercises

Side Neck Stretch

Perform this movement either standing or sitting. With your shoulders even, your feet flat on the floor, and your chin level, look straight ahead. Then gently tilt your head to the right, toward the top of your shoulder, until you feel tension on the left side of the neck and left upper shoulder. Hold this position for a count of ten. Repeat, tilting to the left. Do it twice on each side.

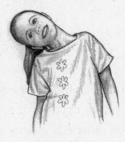

Front Neck Stretch

Perform this movement either standing or sitting. With your shoulders even and your feet flat on the floor, gently tilt your head down, bringing your chin toward your chest until tension is felt in the back of the neck. Hold for fifteen seconds. Repeat only once.

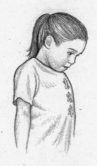

Shoulder Stretch

Perform this movement while either standing or sitting. First, interlock fingers, then raise both arms above the head while turning palms to the ceiling/sky. With palms facing upward and arms extended, gently stretch arms up and back until tension is felt in the shoulder area. Repeat twice.

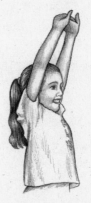

Triceps Stretch

Perform this movement either standing or sitting. With head in an upright position, put your right hand behind your head with your

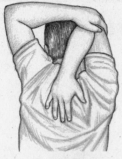

palm touching your left upper shoulder. Place your left hand on top of the elbow of the stretching arm and gently apply light tension to the elbow to stretch the back of the arm. Switch arms, repeat. Do stretch twice more on each side.

Hamstring Stretch

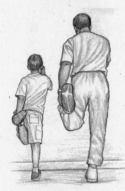

In a standing position, place your left foot slightly in front of the right foot with toe up, heel touching the ground. Next, with upper back straight, bend forward from the waist, lowering your upper body over the left leg until you feel tension in the back of the thigh of the left leg. Switch legs, repeat. Do stretch twice more per leg.

Quad Stretch

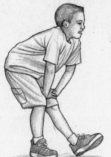

While standing on your right leg, grab the ankle of your left leg and pull your foot up toward your buttock so that you feel tension in the front of your left thigh. Switch legs, repeat. Do stretch twice more per leg.

Back Stretch

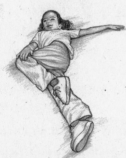

While lying on your back, bend your left leg, placing your left foot alongside your right knee. Next, place your right hand on top of the left knee, gently pushing the knee to the right and in the direction of the floor until you feel tension in the hip and lower back. Keep the upper back and shoulders flat to the floor. Switch sides, repeat. Do stretch twice more on each side.

Calf Stretch
Face a wall and extend your arms half-way so that both hands are pushing against it. Next, place your right foot near the wall and extend your left leg behind you a pace. Gently bend your right knee forward while keeping your left heel flat to the floor and both toes pointing toward the wall. Continue to bend the right knee until you experience light tension in the back of the 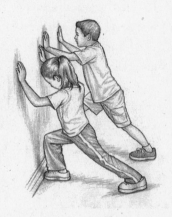 calf (lower leg) of your left leg. Switch legs, repeat. Do stretch twice more per leg.

modeled after adult programs, with strict guidelines and long durations. But kids are more like dragsters than school buses; kids are designed to travel short distances quickly and explosively instead of making long, methodical trips. Children have a lower aerobic capacity compared with adults. In other words, kids tire out much faster than adults when performing long, high-energy activities. I've seen very few kids who enjoy going for a five-mile run, but most children will happily play tag for an hour.

So what's the best way to aerobically train our kids? Take a normal aerobic activity such as walking or jogging and turn it into a game. Instead of jogging for thirty minutes at a time, break the activity up into segments. For instance, challenge your kids to a one-block race. Walk another block, and then challenge them again. Or, instead of telling your kids to swim laps for thirty minutes, put on your swimsuit and try racing them two laps at a time. Let them rest in between.

Interval Training Really Works!

Research supports the benefits of the stop-and-start type of exercises that kids naturally prefer. Interval training has been used for years for developing peak performance in elite endurance athletes. It's been found to improve stamina, muscular strength and endurance, and efficient energy use. In fact, twenty minutes of kid-type, intense, stop-and-start exercise can be equal to, or even have greater benefits than, sixty minutes of adult-type, slow, prolonged walking. Those short bursts of exercise have even been shown to increase growth hormone, which improves muscle, cartilage, and bone growth.

Benefits of aerobic exercise. These vigorous and brisk activities use a lot of oxygen, making you breathe heavier and your heart beat faster. Regular, vigorous aerobic activities strengthen the heart muscles, increase cardiac output and plasma volume, increase respiratory capacity, increase the muscles' ability to store energy, create healthier skin, reduce anxiety and depression, decrease body fat, and strengthen ligaments, tendons, and bone.

Frequency of activity. Encourage your child to do fun active sports or aerobic movements at least three to five days per week for twenty to sixty minutes.

Favorite aerobic activities. If your child already has a favorite sport, great! But if you've got a couch potato, he probably doesn't. You can help your child experiment to find the sport he prefers. (This step is crucial. If you don't help her learn the sport when she starts it, she'll never get good enough to enjoy it.) Let her pick four favorite sports from the list on pages 140–141 and schedule time to practice each with her for one week at a time over the next month. Focus on one activity each week and do that activity with her at least twice during that week.

At the end of the month, talk with your child about which sport she enjoyed the most. Then try to find a local team or class for your child to join. (For the best recommendations, call your school, talk with friends and neighbors, ask your pediatrician, or check at the local YMCA.)

Ask your child to make a commitment to the sport for at least one season (usually two to three months). Explain that the season will be long enough to give him a good idea whether he likes the sport. Take time each day to be the "coach" and practice the sport with him after school.

Remember, the better he is at the sport, the more he will like it and the more he'll want to actively participate. If, after the first season, your child no longer wants to play this sport, just make sure he always has at least one aerobic activity or active sport in his life all the time.

One special note regarding especially heavy children who will be starting physical activities for the first time. *The fatter the child, the slower you need to go with all exercises.* Because an obese child is already carrying around more weight than his sensitive bones and joints can comfortably handle, moving too fast is likely to give your child a case of sore joints or sprains. The advice "walk before you run" is especially true for an obese child trying to get fit. Gradually increase the pace of the walking from slow to brisk to speed walking and then to running. Take months for this progression if that's what your child needs. For muscle building, gradually increase the strength-building exercises or the resistance of the tubing involved. The leaner the child becomes, the easier it will be for him to walk and run faster.

Look at the list of aerobic activities to let your child choose from on pages 140–141.

Beat Boredom

Cross-train to keep it fun. Some kids will happily play basketball every day after school for a couple of hours. Other kids will want to ride a bike or play softball when they're not going to swimming class. Help your children keep their activities as varied as they need to in order to keep them fun.

YOUTHFUL STRENGTH BUILDING

Now that we're more physically active (P), limber (L), and aerobic (A), let's add the finishing touch: "Y"—youthful movements to build stronger muscles. The fourth part of the PLAY Program includes strength-building exercises appropriate for young children, because these exercises help the child use his own body movements as weights. This type of natural resistance is healthier—and more available—than using bulky metal weights. While just moving a muscle is good for it, moving it against resistance (challenging the muscle) is better.

Benefits of youthful strength building. These movements go well beyond just moving the play muscles. They actually *build* more muscle, improve coordination, improve muscle density and tone, and increase energy expenditure during and after movements. They also stimulate growth hormone and insulin growth factors; strengthen bones, ligaments, and tendons; and assist in preventing sports injuries in young athletes. Remember, one of the goals of the LEAN Kids Program is to tone muscle and burn fat—*to make flab firm.* By building more muscle, the "Y" (youthful strength building) raises the resting metabolic rate (the body's fat-burning capability) more than any other part of the LEAN Kids Program.

Frequency of activity. The key to building muscle is consistency. Once you and your child pick the strength-building routine you like (see page 140), it's important that you stick with this every *other* day. Every day is too much; muscles need a day to rest and grow. In fact, it is not during the exercise that your child's muscles grow and become stronger; it is when they are *resting.*

However, if you do your weight-training activities less than twice a week, you may not be challenging muscles enough to grow. We recommend picking a regular schedule (like Monday, Wednesday, and Friday) and a regular time (such as after school) and remembering to *stick with it.* While your child may make the excuse that he doesn't have time to exercise, just remind him that you have time to do it with him.

Once you start formal strength-training exercises, your goal should be to do three to six of them every other day. You and your child should do one set of ten repetitions to start. Build up your strength until you can do two sets of ten each, then more. Take your time to build strength—there's no rush! Remember, "no pain, no gain" is a fallacy. *"No pain, no strain"* is closer to what you're aiming for. Your child should perform each movement slowly and steadily. It should only feel hard (or "burn") during the last two or three movements in a set. Keep it challenging, but keep it fun.

Favorite strengthening exercises. Again, choice is the key to getting your child involved and committed to this activity. And there are lots of different kinds of strength-building exercises your child can choose from. We recommend introducing the most sedentary children to strength building gradually, so we've provided three levels of activities to choose from.

LEVEL ONE—START NATURALLY. You don't have to take your child to a local gym to benefit from strength training. Climbing trees or the playground monkey bars, rock climbing, or even carrying groceries can build strong muscles. You can also use simple household objects such as a soup can or milk container filled with rice or dried beans as weights, as long as they are heavy enough to provide a challenge for your child yet easy enough to grasp.

Any activity that offers resistance to muscles will do. Your child can choose from any of the strength-building exercises listed on page 140.

LEVEL TWO—BUILD GRADUALLY. Once your child is ready to start more formal strength-building activities, let her choose some from the list below.

Heavy Metal Is Not for Young Muscles

The American Academy of Pediatrics and the American Orthopedic Society for Sports Medicine recommend that because of potential injury to their immature bones and muscles, young kids not lift heavy weights for strength training movements without professional supervision.

BODY WEIGHT EXERCISE DESCRIPTIONS

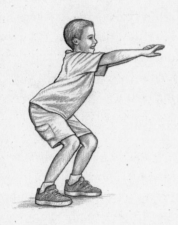

Squat

Place both feet shoulder-width apart, keeping knees slightly bent. Keep your back straight, chin parallel to the floor, shoulders relaxed, and chest up. Bending your knees, slowly lower your weight as if you were sitting in a chair. Pause once you reach a position in which your thighs are roughly parallel to the floor, then slowly stand up while tightening the buttock muscles. Repeat ten times.

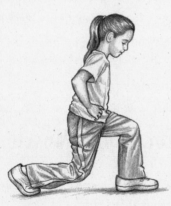

Lunge

Begin with your back straight, chin parallel to the floor, shoulders relaxed and chest up. Step so that one foot is in front of the other by two or three feet (depending on your height). Slowly lower your body down to the floor while leading with the back knee. Keep the front knee in the middle of the foot in the down position. Straighten both legs and return to the start. Repeat ten times per leg.

Side Shoulder Raise

Place feet shoulder-width apart, chin parallel to the floor, back straight, and hands by your side. While maintaining a slight bend in your elbows, slowly raise arms out to the side and up with palms facing the ground. Pause once they have reached shoulder level, then slowly lower them. Repeat ten times.

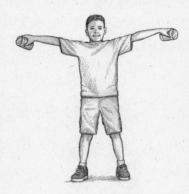

Triceps Extension

Stand with feet shoulder-width apart, knees slightly bent, chin parallel to the floor, with shoulders relaxed. Place the exercising hand behind the head, with elbow bent and angled forward. To begin the movement, slowly extend the exercising arm by raising the hand above the head, keeping the exercising elbow close to the side of the head throughout the entire range of motion. Repeat ten times per arm.

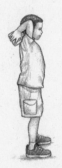

Arm Curls

Place feet shoulder-width apart, chin parallel to the floor, back straight, with your arms lowered by your sides, in line with your shoulders and slightly in front of the hips. Holding a can of soup (or something similar) in each hand, begin your movement by slowly "curling" one forearm up toward your chest while keeping the elbow in front of the hip and the wrist slightly curled up. Tighten your biceps as you bring the forearm up and pause as you reach chest level. Slowly allow the forearm to lower back to the starting position. Repeat ten times for each arm.

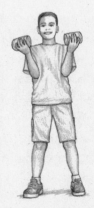

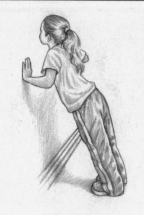

Wall Push-Up
While facing a wall, stand two to three feet away from the wall, raise hands to shoulder height, and place palms against the wall. Keeping back and body straight, lower your body into the wall, bending your elbows. Push your body away from the wall by straightening the arms. Repeat ten times.

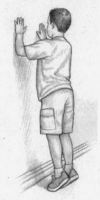

Heel Raises
Placing hands on a wall for support, rise up on the balls of your feet while tightening the lower leg. Repeat ten times.

LEVEL THREE—USE RESISTANCE TUBES! Once you and your child get strong enough, we recommend adding stretch bands (also called resistance bands or tubing) to your PLAY program. These bands or tubes are safer for young muscles and joints than metal weights are. Tubing is available at most sporting goods stores, and they come with instructional brochures and/or videos. (To order, see www.LEANKIDS.com.)

We recommend starting with the following easy exercises. Make sure your beginning bands or tubes are thin and stretchable. As you and your kids gain strength, move on to thicker bands, which will offer more resistance.

Youthful Strength-Building Exercises
Resistance Tube Movements

Lunge

Stand with one foot about two feet in front of the other. Put the front foot on the center of the tubing. Holding a tubing handle in each hand, curl your hands up at shoulder level with elbows down. Keep your back straight, chin parallel to the floor, shoulders relaxed, and chest up. Slowly lower your body weight down to the floor, leading with the back knee. Keep the front knee centered with the front foot. Straighten both legs and return to the start. Repeat ten times.

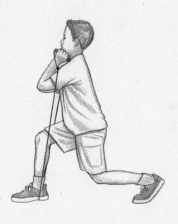

Arm Curl

Place both feet (or one to decrease difficulty) on the center of your tubing, with your feet shoulder-width apart, chin parallel to the floor, and back straight. Lower your arms by your sides, in line with your shoulders and slightly in front of the hips. Holding a tubing handle in each hand, begin your movement by slowly curling the forearms up toward the shoulders while keeping your elbows in front of the hips and your wrists slightly curled up. Tighten your biceps as you bring the forearms up and pause as your hands reach shoulder level. Slowly allow the forearms to lower back to the starting position. Do both arms at the same time or alternate arms. Repeat ten times.

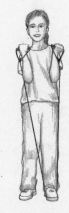

Back Pull

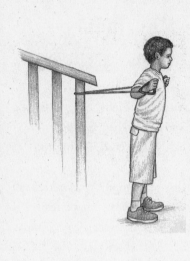

Loop the tubing around a pole. Face away from the pole with your back straight, chin parallel to the floor, shoulders relaxed, and chest up. Holding the tube handles, raise your hands to chest level. Lean forward slightly to create tension on the band, then slowly extend your arms forward. Reach out and in, like you're hugging someone. When arms are fully extended, bring hands together. Slowly release the band back to the start position. Repeat ten times.

Bent Row

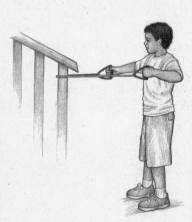

Loop the tubing around a pole so that it can't slip back and forth. Face the pole while holding one tube handle in each hand, arms straight but not locking elbows. Lean backward slightly so there's some tension in the band. Keeping your right arm straight, slowly pull the left hand back underneath your armpit. Then return left arm to the start position with arms straight but not locking your elbow. Repeat motion with the right arm. Repeat motion ten times per arm.

Special tips for strength building. Here are some special tips to help make your strength-building activities as successful and fun as possible.

- **Safety first**. At least at the beginning, an adult should supervise all youthful strength-building movements. Injuries can occur when children are left unsupervised to play with equipment.
- **Don't jerk the joints.** Teach children to lift their bodies or bands *slowly* (especially when beginning a new exercise). Young ligaments, tendons, and joints are easily injured by lifting too much too fast.
- **Learn "how heavy—how often."** It is very important for kids not to begin a program at too high or too low a level. If the resistance is too great, the movement will increase the risk of injury by making it difficult for the child to perform correctly. If the resistance is too low, your child will not experience the gains that he could and may get bored quickly. So if you're using tubing, pick your first set carefully. Your child should be able to do the first five or six movements easily, but strain a little on the last two or three.
- **Start where you need to.** Understand that there will probably be some movements your child may not be able to perform ten times, even with the lightest band. If that's the case, take the time to prepare those muscles. For example, if your child wants to strengthen his upper body, we recommend starting with push-ups. Ask your child to do as many as he can (even if it's only one) slowly and carefully. Just be sure to have him do one every other day, until it's easy. Then have him do two every other day, until that is easy. Start slowly, and as long as you are consistent and do it regularly, your child *will* get stronger.
- **Balance is the buzzword.** Train children to exercise *all* their muscles, not just a few of them. Spot-training (building some muscle groups more than others) may be popular with some adults, but it is not recommended for children. Developing all muscles equally keeps a child's body in balance.

Putting It All Together

Now that you have an understanding of what the PLAY Program is, it's time to put it all together into a personal exercise plan for your child. Here are the next steps I recommend.

PERSONALIZE YOUR PLAY LIST

Below is a chart that lists all the various play, lengthening, aerobic, and youthful strengthening activities we've discussed. Sit down with your child and choose the ones she wants to start with. (Note that the weekly frequency goal is noted at the top of each column.)

Physical Activity	Lengthening Movements	Active Sports/ Aerobic Activities	Strength-Building Movements
Goal: 30–60 minutes per day	*Goal: 3–8 stretches 3–5 days per week*	*Goal: 20–60 minutes 3–5 days per week*	*Goal: 10–30 minutes 3 days per week*
Walk with your family in your neighborhood	Neck stretch	Backpacking	Jungle gym
	Shoulder stretch	Ballet	Rock climbing
	Triceps stretch	Basketball	Tree climbing
Pillow fight with the kids	Hamstring stretch	Cycling	Body weight exercises
	Quad stretch	Dancing	
Throw a Frisbee	Back stretch	Football	Resistance-tube movements
Toss a softball or baseball	Calf stretch	Hiking	
		Gymnastics	
Play a basketball game		Handball	
		Ice skating	
Have a blast with some hula hoops		In-line skating	
		Jogging	
		Martial arts	

Physical Activity	Lengthening Movements	Active Sports/ Aerobic Activities	Strength-Building Movements
Goal: 30–60 minutes per day	*Goal: 3–8 stretches 3–5 days per week*	*Goal: 20–60 minutes 3–5 days per week*	*Goal: 10–30 minutes 3 days per week*
Flip on music and dance Go for a family hike in the country Take the stairs Jump rope with your kids Invite your child to participate in household chores Teach your child to roller skate Play leapfrog, tag, or hide and seek Ride a bike to and from school Garden together Let your child teach a favorite game		Non-impact hockey Racquetball Relay races Rope jumping Rowing Skateboarding Skiing Snorkeling Soccer Softball Stair stepping Swimming Table tennis Tennis Trampoline Volleyball Walking briskly	

LEAN KIDS SAY

"I love the PLAY list! When Dad comes home at night,
we take it out and pick something to do.
It's like a new play adventure every day!"
—DELANEY, AGE EIGHT

TIPS FOR KEEPING IT FUN

Now that you know what to do, we want you to have fun doing it. Here are some tips for making the exercise enjoyable for everyone.

Wear play clothes. Make sure you and your family have appropriate attire for activities, such as walking, cycling, basketball, etc. Wear comfortable shoes that provide support, as well as clothing that is nonrestrictive and breathes well. Once your child shows a commitment to an activity, buy him some of the clothing and equipment specially designed for it. Kids love a "uniform" and it will enhance their enjoyment of the sport.

Keep kids cool. Children, by the very nature of their bodies, are more prone to overheating than adults are during strenuous exercise. Children often don't pay attention to their thirst cues and tend to ignore drinking enough fluids before and during exercise. In addition, prepubertal children don't sweat as much as adults, which causes the body to retain more heat. These quirks in heat-release mechanisms are another reason why short bursts of exercise are physiologically better for children than are long bouts of vigorous exercise.

Exercise right for your type. Whether your child is genetically a banana, apple, pear, or yam, he can enjoy exercise. But a child who matches her activity to her body type and natural skills is more likely to enjoy the activity and stay with it. Of course, I strongly believe that desire is more important than genetic destiny—so don't discourage a child from an interest in a sport, no matter what her body type. But if you want to steer your child toward an activity he might naturally excel in, you'll be interested in these suggestions.

- **Bananas** (genetically lean kids) are slim, lanky fat-burners and tend to carry less body fat. Because slender kids tend to be less muscular, they usually prefer endurance sports, such as long-distance running and track. They tend to be good runners and long-distance swimmers or marathoners. While most banana kids are taller than average and are perfect for sports like basketball and cross-country running, some bananas are petite and can excel in gymnastics.
- **Apples** (kids that are round in the middle) carry more muscle than bananas or pears, so they tend to excel at strength-related activities, such as wrestling and football.
- **Pears** (kids who are thicker below the waist) have a higher fat-to-muscle ratio than apples or bananas. Because this type tends to store fat in the lower half of their bodies, a pear is unlikely to run a four-minute mile, yet could very well excel in martial arts and short-distance endurance sports.
- **Yams** (kids who are just plain big from top to bottom) tend to be strong as children. They excel at power sports, like football, basketball, and rugby.

11 Tips for Selecting the Proper Athletic Shoe

One of the most important items you can purchase to help your child's PLAY experience be successful is a good pair of athletic shoes. Poorly fitted athletic shoes can lead to problems such as sore heels, lower back pain, ingrown toenails, corns, fatigue, sore muscles, and poor posture. These problems can be avoided by following some of these simple tips.

1. Try to purchase shoes toward the end of the day, when your child's feet are most swollen.

2. Go to a reputable shoe store where your child can try on athletic shoes. Be sure the store has knowledgeable salespeople who can help you fit the shoe properly.

3. Bring in your child's old shoes and have the salesperson take a look at them. Frequently he will be able to tell if your child's feet supinate (roll out a little) or pronate (roll inward) just by looking at the wear and tear on your kid's shoes.

4. Because kids' feet change so fast, have your child's feet measured for width and length every time you buy new shoes.

5. Make sure that your child tries on both shoes, in case each foot is a different size.

6. When purchasing shoes, make sure that your child wears the same type of socks she plans to wear with the shoes. Your child's toes should be able to wiggle freely.

7. Look for a shoe that provides adequate cushioning and support. You might even want to purchase *heel cushions* (available at pharmacies or shoe stores) for children over eight. Remember to try your new shoes on *with* the pad inside. I recommend heel cushions for overweight children of any age.

8. If your child has flat feet or pronates, look into having *orthotic inserts* made for your child.

9. Cross-trainers are a great choice for all types of play. But if your child is committed to one sport, buy a specialized shoe. Running, basketball, tennis, baseball, and soccer all have special shoes.

10. Kids can grow out of shoes in a few months, so be sure and check how their feet are feeling. Old shoes can cause injuries, so check for signs of wear and replace the shoes when necessary.

11. Be prepared to spend more for a quality shoe. A bargain shoe that causes blisters and other foot problems is really no bargain.

MOTIVATING KIDS TO MOVE

All these health benefits may convince you that exercise is worth the effort, but they probably won't motivate your nine-year-old. And while all of these activities look great on paper, most parents want to know how they can use the PLAY Program to get kids to move more during the course of their day. As with other parts of the LEAN Kids Program, getting started is usually the hardest part. Once kids start exercising, they'll probably enjoy it enough to keep it up on their own.

So here are some ideas for how to get them started.

Start slow and work up gradually. Especially if your child has been inactive until now, be sure to start slowly. Don't leap into the soccer league. Start by taking twenty-minute walks together every day. Gradually build up to hour-long walks. Take things one step at a time. If a sport is hard, it's not fun, and your child will resist. If you keep each step easy enough to master, your child will enjoy his success and want to continue.

Work out while you watch TV. This is a great way to introduce kids to exercise almost without their even noticing. Most young children are fidgety when they watch TV; it's actually hard for them to sit still for the hours that they watch. Keep exercise equipment (like home gym equipment, hula hoops, mini-trampolines, Twister, Resist-a-Balls, and jump ropes, or just your resistance bands) in the TV room. During an hour of television, two minutes of medium-intensity exercise done during each of the five commercial breaks could translate into as much as five pounds of extra fat burned per year. Easy commercial-break exercises: toe lifts, heel lifts, squats, and lunges. Better yet, park your exercise bike there and wait until your child asks to use it. Don't worry, he will! Once the kids start using and enjoying these moving opportunities, introduce the "screen time equals moving time" rule.

Screen time equals moving time. I've referred to this rule a few times in this book, but let me take this opportunity to fully explain it. We have an exercise rule in the Sears home that we call "screen time equals moving time." For every minute of screen time the child indulges in, she must also move for one minute in some type of physical activity.

That activity can be formal exercise or just walking around. If she wants an hour of screen time at the TV or computer, she can have it only after she has finished the physical activity. You don't have to keep an exact time log, and remember to include the routine moving that your kids do during the course of their day (walking to school, climbing stairs, doing chores) as well as the more formal exercises they embark on. The rule sounds scary at first to a lot of kids, but you can show them how quickly their moving time adds up—and how it might be so much fun to do that they won't even want as much screen time as they earn!

Invite your child to take a walk with you. She'll love the attention so much that she might not notice she's exercising. And don't just walk. Use that time to talk, laugh, share your day. Your child will treasure the time and associate exercise with those good feelings.

Pedometers for Little Pedestrians

Kids love to compete with themselves. A handy device that I find helpful to motivate little movers is a pedometer, a matchbox-size gadget that clips onto a belt, pants, or skirt waist and records the number of steps taken each day. When children enroll in our LEAN Kids Program, I instruct them on how to use a pedometer and how to construct a progress chart. For the habitual sitter, 5,000 steps a day is an achievable beginning goal; for the medium mover, 10,000 steps a day; and for the "love to move" child, 20,000 steps a day. Each day (or on a weekly average), have the child plot on a chart the number of steps he took. Plotting the pedometer steps helps the child visualize her progress. Children love to play "beat the numbers" games.

Think of a family hobby that requires lots of movement. When Martha and I took up swing dancing, our teens did, too. Many families enjoy biking, skiing, or swimming together. You'll see a

Pedometer Chart

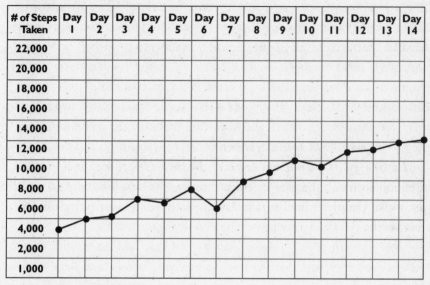

# of Steps Taken	Day 1	Day 2	Day 3	Day 4	Day 5	Day 6	Day 7	Day 8	Day 9	Day 10	Day 11	Day 12	Day 13	Day 14
22,000														
20,000														
18,000														
16,000														
14,000														
12,000														
10,000														
8,000														
6,000														
4,000														
2,000														
1,000														

Goal: >10,000 steps a day

list of suggested sports activities on pages 140–141. Look for one you can do as a family. Get your kids going.

Choose active friends. Invite other families to join you for an afternoon of fun and games. Arrange play dates in the park, not in front of the television.

Play King for the Week

A lean parent told me, "Each week our kids rotate who's going to be our PLAY leader who plans the activities for the week. The leader also takes everyone through the different movements we do as a family. Our seven-year-old daughter, Julie, loves to be the PLAY leader for the week and to correct all of us when we are doing our movements wrong!"

Let your child choose. I've tried to emphasize throughout this chapter how important it is to let your child choose his own activities. Offer a wide variety of options, and let your child pick what she wants to try first. Some children might love a team sport like baseball or football, but other children prefer solitary forms of exercise, like swimming or running. More cerebral children often enjoy martial arts, which is a terrific confidence builder. The point is that the more you let your child express herself through her physical activity, the more she'll enjoy it.

You make all the difference. If your kid is not athletically inclined or keen on joining a team, take the time to play with him yourself. The more practice he gets in kicking a soccer ball or catching a baseball with you, the better he'll get. You might find he builds the confidence to join the school team after all.

Play with your kids. Play tag or ball or Frisbee, ride bikes, roller-skate, and participate in pool games, yard games, and park games. *We believe that the family who plays together stays lean together!* Need some ideas? Try these after-school games with your kids. (You'll be surprised how enjoyable and relaxing they are for you, too.)

FOLLOW THE LEADER. Do movements such as push-ups, jumping jacks, or jogging in place. Try lunging along with fun hand movements. Your child will follow along with you.

PLAY SIMON SAYS. Again, use movements from your own exercise routine for the command of "Simon Says." For example, "Simon says, stretch your hamstring" or "Simon says, stretch your arms and reach for the ceiling with your fingertips." If you're not familiar with a variety of stretches, just use some of the ones we showed you in the Play and Lengthening sections on pages 125–129.

"MOTHER/FATHER, MAY I?" If you have more than one child, ask them to line up approximately fifty feet away from you. Instruct them to take turns doing bunny hops or lunges to advance toward you by making requests with the phrase, "Mother/Father, may I?" For example, "Mother, may I do five big bunny hops?" or "Father, may I take ten lunge steps?" The child can move only if you reply, "Yes, you may." The object of the game is to be the first child to reach you, which will inspire your kids to jump and lunge as far as they can!

Plan time for PLAY. If you don't plan it, it's probably not going to happen! That's true of most important things in our lives, isn't it? We encourage you to set a scheduled time for the PLAY program. Try asking your kids every day after school what PLAY activity they'd like to spend thirty minutes on. Schedule one weekend day each week for a family activity. Sign up for a sport once a week, so that you have a class to attend that you can't skip. Feel like you don't have time? When parents in my practice say that, I tell them they have a choice. They can make thirty to sixty minutes a day to move with their kids today—or reserve more time for the hospital later. The PLAY program is good for you, too!

Use a weekly planner. In order to organize your efforts to exercise more, you might want to use this weekly planner. Just make copies and fill them out with your children. They will enjoy charting their progress. It often inspires children to try harder in the coming week.

	Monday	Tuesday	Wednesday	Thursday	Friday	Saturday	Sunday
Play							
Lengthening exercises							
Aerobics							
Youthful strengthening							

Moving More Is a Lifelong Habit

We hope this chapter has left you with a ton of ideas for how to get your child started on a more active way of living—today! As you get your child moving, realize that besides building young muscle, you're shaping young minds. By teaching and training your child to value a toned, healthy body, you're building a mind-set, a lifelong habit in which your child grows up enjoying the look and feel of a lean body.

8

ATTITUDE

Think Lean

When it comes to success and happiness in life, it's all about attitude. By attitude, we simply mean the outward expression of inward feelings. In the LEAN Kids Program, we recognize that feeling good—healthier and stronger—helps ensure a good attitude. Getting lean is part of getting happy.

The LEAN Kids Program helps the child have a good attitude about health and, above all, value his body. As I stated in *The Successful Child*, I believe a positive attitude is one of the best success tools you can give your child. Remember, the LEAN Kids Program is not only a wellness program for the body, it is also a fitness program for the mind. The mind and body are intimately related; what's good for one is good for the other. Not only will the LEAN Kids Program help your children build leaner bodies, it will help them build leaner minds.

Think of the LEAN Kids Program as a gardening tool that helps your child's developing mind weed out and prune thoughts and habits that weigh it down, while feeding its soil with nutrients that help its flowers bloom. Now let's look at how to help your child get an "A" in attitude.

The Biochemistry of Attitude

The LEAN Kids Program helps regulate your child's level of happy hormones (serotonin, endorphins, dopamine, and norepinephrine), which are secreted by the pituitary gland, the pea-sized master gland located deep within the base of the brain. Happy hormones regulate mood, appetite, sleep, and general well-being. (See chapter 4 for more on hormones.) When they get out of balance, they contribute to depression, anxiety, and many other mood disorders. Prozac and other mood-regulating medicines work by increasing the levels of the happy hormones, especially serotonin.

Using the LEAN Kids Program is like *self-medicating* the brain—without the unpleasant side effects of factory-made mood elevators. Self-medicating is best, especially for growing children, because it *appropriately* stimulates happy hormones—just the right amount, at the right time, and in optimal balance.

The more balanced your hormones, the happier you feel. Just how does the LEAN Kids Program work this magic? Here are some strategies you can teach your child so that he can intentionally balance and boost his happy hormones.

Fat Is Not Happy

Studies show that obese people tend to have lower levels of happy hormones, or endorphins.

MOVE TO BOOST HAPPY HORMONES

Besides helping to lean off excess fat, exercise releases happy hormones, especially serotonin and endorphins. Because exercise jogs the release of happy hormones, teach your child that when he feels sad he should get moving. Studies show that bouts of repetitive activities, such as walking or riding a bicycle or stationary bike, can elevate levels of happy hormones. Even kid habits like fidgeting and chewing gum may be a child's instinctive way of relaxing, since these activities can also stimulate happy hormones. Wise parents can help fidgety children by offering to go outside and play with them.

FEED THE HAPPY HORMONES

Feed your child "happy meals"—no, not the McDonald's kind. The very act of eating releases serotonin, which contributes to the pleasure of dining.

How certain foods affect mood varies from child to child. Some kids go squirrelly after downing a frozen syrupy drink; others don't seem bothered. Keep your child's personal food-mood diary. Carbohydrates tend to affect moods, for better or worse. A right-carb diet (discussed in the nutrition chapter) tends to be a happy meal. Right carbs with the right combinations of other foods seem to be the happiest meals. Right carbs stimulate the release of happy hormones, especially serotonin, in the right way—a slow, steady elevation.

Wrong carbs (like the sugar in soda and sweet snacks) stimulate serotonin in the wrong way—a huge, happy elevation followed by a big, sad crash. Too much sugar too fast bothers the brain.

Lean Lesson: Good food equals good mood!

Heavy meals are not so happy. A large, high-carb meal can be sedating, which is okay for dinner but not for breakfast or lunch on a school day. A brainy breakfast combines complex carbs with some protein and healthy fats. A high-protein lunch can temporarily boost mental acuity, but a large lunch high in fat or carbs can increase the afternoon sluggishness that schoolchildren often experience.

LAUGH TO INCREASE HAPPY HORMONES

Try to be a funny family. Laughter can lighten up a serious child and cheer up a sad child. Sometimes when you've just had a bad day or you really messed up, just hug your child, put on a smile, and say, "Let's take some time out and sit down and watch a funny movie together." The message you're giving your child is, "Let's lighten up."

Laughter is like a humorous aerobic workout. It increases heart rate and blood circulation, followed by an after-laugh relaxed state. While it's true that you can worry yourself sick, you can also laugh yourself well.

Food Is Not a Happiness Pill

While eating a healthful meal can make us feel satisfied and even raise our hormone levels to make us feel happy, food itself should not be mistaken for a happiness tool. Be careful about sabotaging a healthy attitude about food by using it to reward good behavior, or withdrawing it as a punishment. I've seen so many parents comfort a crying child by saying, "Here, have a drink of your soda" or "Have a bite of your cookie" to make him feel better. While that strategy usually works because it distracts the child from his discomfort, it also gives children a terrible message about eating food for emotional rather than nutritional reasons. When your children feel sad, give them a hug and a smile. It's better for them!

Studies show a direct relationship between a joyful attitude and recovery from serious illness.

Laughter lowers stress hormones and raises the happy hormones. Besides helping children have a cheerful attitude, laughter helps them stay well by boosting the level of immunoglobulins and natural killer white blood cells, the body's own antibiotics.

Laughter is the body's best relaxation technique. A hearty belly laugh involves the work of many muscles in the face, abdomen, and diaphragm, a humorous workout that diverts attention from tense muscles elsewhere in the body.

Yet boosting and balancing hormones is not the only way the LEAN Kids Program can help give your child a healthy attitude. Let's talk about some of the other techniques you can use.

Help Children Like Their Bodies

When ten-year-old Jason came into my office for obesity counseling, he didn't like his body. And since he disliked the reflection he saw in the mirror, he didn't like himself.

Kids are honest mirrors. Unlike many adults, they don't fake what they feel. Jason appeared sad because he *was* sad. The cycle of obesity created a cycle of unhappiness. Because he was fat, he flopped in flag football. Kids teased him, which caused him to sit on the sidelines and stew—and get fatter. His anger gave him an unpleasant attitude, which made him more unpleasant to be around, which caused the other kids to shun him, which made him more angry, which left him more alone, which made him more fat. He didn't like himself because he perceived that other kids didn't like him.

In our first meeting I didn't say to Jason, "I'm going to help you lose weight" (which would only emphasize to Jason that something was wrong with his body). Instead, I opened our discussion with "Jason, I want to help you be able to run faster and to really like your body." His face turned from sad to glad. There was a happy kid inside, buried under his belief that he didn't fit into the crowd.

Helping a fat child like his body when the media applauds thinness requires sensitive parenting. Obviously, the child perceives that something is different about his body, because otherwise he wouldn't be going to a fat counselor or Mom wouldn't be reading this book. You can't just lie to your kids and tell them they're okay. Try these like-your-body attitude adjusters instead.

LIKE YOUR BODY TYPE

As we've discussed, it's important when you talk to your child about health not to imply that one body type is better than another. This can be tricky because children usually perceive thin people as more attractive than robust ones. But remind them that some of their strongest sports figures aren't thin. Moreover, if you have a daughter or son interested in sports, look for other role models who are lean and strong. Here are some other ideas for helping your child build a positive attitude toward her own body.

PRAISE YOUR CHILD'S BODY

Instead of focusing on your child's fatness, point out her attractive qualities. Does she have a nice voice? Does he have a pleasant smile or strong arms? Is her hair pretty? Drop these like-your-body messages whenever the opportunity arises.

Obese children get the message, "I'm klutzy and ungraceful." Often their schoolmates mock their clumsiness. Remember, children measure themselves by how they believe others perceive them. Offer an occasional "nice move" when she's dancing, kicks a soccer ball, or performs another physical activity.

FRAME GOOD FEELINGS

"Framing" refers to how your child perceives that you (or others) view her. Positive framing (viewing your child positively) is the foundation of Self-image Building 101. If parents (and other significant people in a child's life) frame the child in a positive way, the child is more likely to have a positive attitude about himself.

For instance, if somebody says, "She's so fat" in front of your daughter, counteract that negative feedback with positive framing. Point out that she's also very funny and gets top grades at school. But framing doesn't mean lying to your kids. If your child says, "I'm fat," don't discount her feelings. Instead, make this comment a teachable moment to help her get lean, if she needs to. Then immediately switch the topic to her success skills. Remind her, "You sure are a good soccer player," or whatever her special skill is.

Raise a Positive Child

You've heard the advice, "Set your mind to it." That's what you're doing when you program a child's developing brain with positive beliefs instead of negative ones. Attitudes are contagious, especially from parents to children. Your child will inherit the attitudes shared by your family because it's what she perceives as the norm.

That's why it's so important to model optimism. The more positive you can be, the more positive your kids will be. And I don't mean just smiling all the time. You can't fool your kids when you're sad inside. Yet, you can show them that you can cope with troubles, and remain optimistic while you do so.

Don't Worry, Live Longer

The expression "worried to death" has a physiological basis. Anxious people who worry more die sooner (usually from heart disease) than do persons who are able to manage their stress. Research shows that optimists, compared with pessimists, tend to live healthier and longer lives.

NURTURE A POSITIVE ATMOSPHERE

Whenever you're with your child, look for teachable moments to model a positive attitude. If you're driving along and you see a demolished car but no ambulances, you might comment, "Thank God no one is hurt."

If he is bummed over losing a soccer game, cheer him up by saying, "Yes, but your team is getting better and you blocked some great shots!" Better yet, be alert to positive statements your child may make on his own, and support them. "We lost the baseball game, but I was glad I got to pitch" deserves a response such as, "Yes, and you pitched really well today."

Also, model a positive attitude for her. If your beloved boss announces one day that he is leaving to take a different job, don't complain about it to your kids. Instead, point out that "while I'm sure I'll miss him, because I learned a lot from him, I'm looking forward to the new things I'll learn from my new boss."

"TEN THINGS TO LIKE"

An attitude accelerator I have used successfully for children who have a poor self-image is to have them list "Ten things I like about me." I ask them to post this list in a place where they'll see it every day, such as their bedroom door, and look at it when they get up in the morning. Then I encourage the kids to add to the list as they begin liking more things about themselves—which they do as their own personal LEAN Kids Program progresses. (See related charts on pages 226–228 and 229.)

THANK GOD!

Some ancient religions have a saying: "Thank God one hundred times each day." Whatever your family's beliefs are, throughout your day let your child hear as many "Thank God" positives as you can.

TURN PROBLEMS INTO OPPORTUNITIES

While being overweight and not physically fit is a problem, it's also an opportunity. In the journey to becoming lean, children will learn more about their bodies and about good nutrition than they knew before. They'll enjoy more time with you. And, if they stick with the program, they'll enjoy their success. A valuable tool for life is to teach your children to turn problems into opportunities.

Edison saw darkness as an opportunity to invent the lightbulb. Instead of focusing on being fat, help your children become excited about becoming lean. The more they can enjoy the daily progress and victories they achieve on the LEAN Kids Program, the more they will have a head start on principles of health and happiness that can last a lifetime.

"Oh, it's raining today. Well, instead of our picnic, we'll make cookies. I've wanted to have an afternoon for cookie baking!" One afternoon when my children were young, I promised to take them to a movie. When we got to the theater, it turned out that the show times had changed and we had missed the movie we had selected. "Let's go for a walk instead." We ended up finding a new toy store to visit and a restaurant that was so good that it became one of their favorites. "You never know," I reminded them.

Teach your child to turn lemons into lemonade. A success tool I try to teach my children is, "You seldom can control circumstances, but you can always control your reaction to them." Throughout life, your children will encounter many misfortunes, and how they react to life's setbacks can mean the difference between an enriching or a defeating experience. If your child is bummed because she hurt her leg and had to quit the soccer team, you might remind her that she now has time to decorate her room, which she always wanted to do. And she can rejoin the team when she's better. Help her to not dwell on what she lost, but look for what she's gaining. Mood-switching strategies are valuable success tools for life.

When I was recovering from cancer, I studied many research articles on the characteristics of survivors, or people who overcame serious mental and physical problems associated with cancer to become stronger than they were before. Why did they survive? The pattern I noticed is that survivors *studied their problem*, became *expert* in it, and used their knowledge *to develop* their personal wellness program; then they eventually *shared* their knowledge with others.

So, it's important that you don't just tell your children what to eat and what exercises to do. Instead of dictating orders to your child, share the knowledge you've gained from the LEAN Kids Program. They need to understand it to know it and live it. Once it's their own, they'll have the gift of health, strength, and happiness for life.

In other words, turn the problem of their overfatness and underfitness into a family project to learn more about nutrition and exercise, and to design a new lifestyle filled with healthy habits.

THE ART OF MENTAL U-TURNS

We all feel bad when life isn't good. Often, the feelings are worse than the circumstances that caused them. When a negative thought enters the brain, it's like a smoker entering a sealed room. The smoke will gradually pollute the air unless you open a window or extinguish the cigarette.

Help your child avoid toxic thoughts that can escalate into a mind full of negative feelings. I call these mental U-turns, or rewind messages. When a toxic thought enters your mind and you feel your thoughts head in a negative direction, start again with more positive thinking. Tell your child that when her head fills with sad or scary thoughts, she can say, "Get out of my head, you worry thought. I don't need you."

Our family hobby is sailing, and we often charter a boat in the Caribbean for our family vacation. Part of the fun of boating is that something usually goes wrong and needs fixing. One day our engine died and we limped under sail into a marina on a remote island, hoping to find a mechanic to fix us up. We were all worried that the situation would ruin our plans, but we were greeted by a friendly mechanic who said, "No problem, mon!" Everyone relaxed. We ended up enjoying the time we spent on that island and learned some lessons about Caribbean life while the locals fixed our boat.

Helping Others Helps Yourself

Help the less fortunate. By making someone else happy, you make yourself happy. Do volunteer work—with your child—to help those less fortunate than you.

FOCUS ON THE SOLUTION

Whenever possible, if your child comes to you with a problem, respond, "Let's find a way to fix it." That response gives your child the important message that it's human to mess up. Rather than getting bogged down with regret, encourage them to face their situation head-on by taking responsibility for the problem and immediately looking for a solution. And remember not to spend time reprimanding them, especially if they realize their mistake. Show them that the point is to fix a problem, not lay blame for it.

PLAY DOWN SMALLIES

Instead of wasting energy worrying, children need to use their energy for growing. Early on, teach them not to clutter their mind with worries about small problems, or what I call "smallies." Smallies are life's little annoyances that merit less than a minute of worry. Your child is riding his tricycle and falls. He's not hurt, but the tricycle is dented. "That's a smallie," you explain. "Glad you weren't hurt!"

Explain to your child that he should save his energy and worry for "biggies," those problems that are more than little annoyances. Biggies might require more creative thinking to turn them into opportunities.

Wash Worry Thoughts Away

I've always thought that negative thoughts are like footprints in the sand. Allow the surf of positive thoughts to come in and wash them away immediately. If you don't, your sand will turn to concrete, and those negative footprints could last forever and become part of your brain.

Teach Your Child How to Relax

One of the most valuable tools for healthy living is the ability to relax. Stress is a fact of life. We can't avoid it, so the best thing we can do for our children is teach them how to deal with it.

It's hard to explain stress to your child, but she'll probably understand if you say, "Too much stress can leave you feeling tense, so your muscles hurt, and your mind is all confused." One of my patients said, "I know what you mean! Sometimes my head gets all in a jambles!" Explain that relaxing is all about untangling those jumbled feelings. Relaxing is feeling good when the world around you doesn't seem so good.

RELAXATION BOOSTS HAPPY HORMONES

Feeling stressed means that you've exhausted your brain's supply of natural happy hormones, so you don't feel good and can't think clearly. Relaxation allows your happy hormones to recuperate from the exhaustion created by stress. Try these following relaxation techniques, which you can describe to your child as "stress busters."

You Can Change Your Brain

New technology is showing that you can actually change your brain by changing your thoughts. PET (positron-emission tomography) scans have detected changes in neuroactivity in the brain in response to happy thoughts. These landmark neurochemistry studies suggest that filling the brain with happy thoughts (called positive self-talk) may create a generally positive brain by building more positive brain circuits than negative ones. On the other hand, filling the mind with unhappy thoughts (negative self-talk) can fill the brain with negative circuitry. This positive brain-building effect is magnified while the brain is still growing in childhood. Concerning brain programming, there's a motto: "Neurons that fire together, wire together." The attitude-building part of the LEAN Kids Program is basically helping the growing brain make the right connections.

ENCOURAGE MINI-MEDITATIONS

Mini-meditations are a few minutes of time-out to clear the mind in the midst of our busy days. Meditation clears the mind of stressors and helps the calming biochemicals or happy hormones to overcome the unhappy ones.

The form of meditation that works best with children uses *mental imagery*. Help your children fill their minds with pleasant thoughts, such as replaying fun scenes, ball games, vacations, and happy relationships with friends. Explain that when they feel upset or frazzled, they should take three deep breaths, close their eyes, and take a minute to think about something that makes them feel good. Maybe it's a place, a person, a stuffed toy, or a hug from you. Whatever they prefer, tell them to designate it as their calming pal and use it for mini-meditations throughout the day.

TAKE A DEEP BREATH

Breathing is key to relaxation. When anxious, we tend to click into shallow chest breathing. To counteract this, most children need to be shown how to breathe correctly.

The phrase "take a deep breath" is anatomically correct. Teach your child to take a long, slow breath that first fills his lungs and then pushes his tummy out. This allows all the breathing muscles to expand and let the most air in. Relaxation specialists call this "breathing with awareness." By increasing the amount of oxygen your body absorbs and helping to balance the body's biochemistry, you reduce stress anxiety.

When children are aware of the mechanics of taking a deep breath, they can always use it to help calm themselves. Play show-and-tell: Show your child how to put her hand above her belly button and feel her abdomen getting bigger as she takes a deep breath and to count slowly to four as she feels her hand moving out. If your child needs more help, add a bit of imagery: "When you slowly breathe out, feel all the tenseness leaving your body through your toes, like honey spilling out of a jar."

PLAY MUSIC

Music mellows the mind. While admittedly some rock and rap music is less than relaxing, the right kind of music can help a child's mind get into the right mood by releasing the happy hormone endorphins.

We play lots of classical music in our home. When our children asked why, we explained, "It helps us relax." Maybe you don't like classical music. Many kinds of music can help you relax. When your child is tense, play the music that helps *you* relax. Ask him if it helps him feel calm. If it does, you might consider giving him music lessons. Making music is even more powerful as a relaxation tool than listening to it.

A HUMAN TOUCH

Especially if your child is the touchy-feely type, give her a brief mini-massage or a long back rub when she is stressed. The skin (the largest organ of the body) is richly supplied with nerves that when stimulated, as during massage, can encourage the brain to release happy hormones. For some kids, this is the best path to calmness.

Here's to a Happy Child

A child cannot be considered truly healthy unless he is happy, too. While most children will grow happier as they make the fitness and nutritional habits of the LEAN Kids Program their own, happiness is not something we can take for granted. Our children need our love and support every day. I hope this chapter has given you some practical tools for helping your children have a positive joyful outlook on life and toward themselves.

9

NUTRITION

What to Eat

Kids seldom get fat from eating too much; they get fat from eating the wrong foods. The LEAN Kids Program's nutritional guidelines are not about calorie counting; they are about learning to make healthy food choices a habit for your child. We designed the LEAN Program to shape your child's tastes, to give her a head start in becoming lean for life.

In this first chapter on lean nutrition, we'll talk about lean choices you can teach your child to make. Your job as your child's lean eating coach is to share the important lessons in this chapter with your child so that she understands why these choices are good for her. Once we review what to eat in this chapter, we'll talk about how and when to eat in chapter 10. By the time you're done with both chapters, your child will be enjoying nutritional food more, feel better after eating, and realize the true meaning of "health foods."

As your child's coach, you need to know how to be your family's home nutritionist. We want you to fully understand and appreciate the healthfulness of lean eating so that your whole family becomes passionate about this program. So let's get started.

Lean Choice #1: Eat "Grow" Foods

What I call "grow" foods are those that are rich in the nutrients that help young bodies thrive. They don't have empty calories, meaning energy without nutritional content. Instead, they have calories that are full of the vitamins and minerals our children need to grow and be strong.

Grow foods are good for overeaters because they are more filling, prompting these children to naturally eat less. Grow foods are good for apparent undereaters ("picky eaters") because they pack lots of nutrition into a small volume.

GROW FOODS GROW HEALTHIER KIDS

What are grow foods? They are whole foods, or foods that have been only minimally processed. They include all fresh fruits and vegetables, all whole grains, all nuts, all lean meats, all legumes, all lean dairy products, and all deep-sea fish (see the grow foods list, page 167).

That's a lot of food! Everyone can find foods they like on a list like this. And the best part is that children seldom get fat from eating too much of any of these foods.

If you think the list will be too hard to remember, just keep this Golden Rule in mind: *The closer a food is to its original form and the less packaged it is, the better it is for your child.* Whole foods help your whole child grow.

Organic Is Best

What about organic foods? They're better for you and your child. This is especially true of dairy products and meats, which are otherwise exposed to antibiotics and steroids whose effect on your child is unclear. Organic fruits and vegetables are better, too, and the thinner their skin, the more important it is that they're organic. You can think of the peel, skin, and shell of foods as a protective shield—the thicker they are, the fewer pesticides and pollutants get to the food itself. Also, it's nearly impossible to scrub all the pesticides off a strawberry, blackberry, or raspberry. If you can't buy organic fruits and vegetables, be sure to wash them with soap and water before consuming them.

TEACH KIDS ABOUT GROW FOODS

I like to introduce children to the concept of grow foods with the Golden Rule above because it's easy for them to grasp. You'll need to know more about grow foods to live the LEAN Kids Program.

For instance, some fish is better than others—we recommend salmon, tuna, and other fish rich in omega-3 oils. In addition, some meats are better for you than others (you always want the leanest cuts possible).

What's even more important is that you thoroughly understand the concept of why whole foods are better for you than packaged foods. And it's not a difficult concept to grasp! Just look at the ingredient labels on packaged food. All those chemicals—and corn syrup—are not good! Show your child the ingredient list on a popular breakfast cereal. Now show him the ingredient list on an apple. There isn't one! He'll get the point pretty quickly.

The Cost of Eating Lean

You may think, "Organic food costs too much!" The fact is that nonorganic food ultimately costs more. Nowhere is it truer that "you get what you pay for." Packaged foods and fast foods may seem cheap, but that's because they're less than they seem. Organic foods are also safer. I'm amazed at how many parents will fork out three dollars for a cup of coffee, yet they shun paying an extra dollar for organic produce or wild instead of farmed fish. You'll get more bang for your buck by buying whole foods rather than packaged ones. If you do the preparation yourself, you can save money *and* keep the junk out. Finally, if none of that convinces you, keep this in mind: The reality is that you can pay for healthful food now—or pay the doctor later. By the time you factor in the extra medical costs related to a junk-food diet—more illnesses, more missed school and work-days—paying more for better food is a smarter investment.

THE LEAN KIDS GROW FOOD LIST

With these concerns in mind, we've developed a specific list of grow foods. To earn a position on our grow foods list, a food must meet one or more of the following criteria:

- it must be nutrient dense (packing the most nutrients per calorie)
- it must be fiber-rich and filling
- it must contribute to balanced blood-sugar levels
- it must be free of food colorings and hydrogenated oils

GREEN-LIGHT GROW FOODS

- Almonds
- Apples
- Artichokes
- Avocados
- Beans (especially lentils and chickpeas)
- Beef
- Blueberries
- Broccoli
- Canola oil
- Cantaloupe
- Carrots
- Chicken
- Chili peppers
- Cranberries
- Eggs
- Fish, especially salmon and tuna
- Flax oil
- Flaxseeds (ground)
- Garlic
- Grapefruit, pink
- Grapes, red
- Leafy greens, spinach
- Mangos
- Olive oil
- Onions
- Oranges
- Papaya
- Peanut butter
- Rice, wild
- Soybeans and tofu
- Sunflower seeds
- Sweet potatoes
- Tomatoes
- Turkey
- Walnuts
- Watermelon
- Whole grains
- Yogurt

Share this grow food chart with your child. You might even want to post it on your refrigerator. Encourage your child to refer to this list when he's looking for a snack. Help her to make grow food choices by having these foods readily available in your home for snacking and incorporating them regularly in your meals.

Veggie Tips

Okay, you know your child needs to eat more vegetables, but how can you make them more attractive for your child to eat? As any marketing expert will tell you, it's all how you package it. Here are some veggie tips from the Sears' family kitchen:

Dip it. Dip sliced raw vegetables into refried beans, guacamole, a pumpkin or squash dip, tomato sauce or paste, and hummus.

Top it. Put your favorite tomato sauce over steamed veggies.

Hide it. Slip grated or diced veggies into favorite foods, such as brown or wild rice, macaroni and cheese, and other pasta dishes. Chances are she'll like the favorite so much that she'll readily accept the veggies that tag along.

Design it. Make veggie art. Create colorful plate faces with tomato ears, olive-slice eyes, a carrot nose, a bell-pepper mustache, and a guacamole beard. Our children loved zucchini pancakes with pea eyes, a carrot nose, shredded cheese hair, and a green bean smile.

Flavor it. If your child perceives vegetables as bland, perk up the flavor with seasonings, such as a dash of salt, lemon juice, honey, dill, cinnamon, or nutmeg. Raisins add a sweet taste to salads and stir-frys. Here's how to make our favorite dish: steam swiss chard, then stir-fry these greens in olive oil with raisins, walnuts, and garlic.

Ketch it. One of our children was addicted to ketchup. Rather than get into the hassle of getting rid of the ketchup, we simply served a healthier ketchup, so at least he would get more tomatoes than sugar. Buy ketchup that is sweetened with fruit concentrate instead of sugar or corn syrup. Try "ketch-oil." Mix a tablespoon of flax oil with three tablespoons of ketchup. Stir well. Use it as a spread or dip.

Pizza it. Veggie pizza is a likely favorite for most kids.

Slurp it. Make soup with a variety of chunky vegetables. Try chili with kidney beans and black beans and vegetarian chili made with soy chunks instead of meat. Lentil soup is our family favorite.

Stir it. With your child, make a vegetable stir-fry and let her choose beef, tofu (firm), chicken, or seafood as her favorite accompaniment.

Cover it. Cover up the evidence. Camouflage new foods with old favorites. Smother the new veggie burger with your child's favorite condiments. Our ten-year-old ate several "burgers" before she discovered we made the healthier switch.

Egg it. Stuff diced veggies into a cheese (parmesan is the most nutritious) omelet. Try: onions, tomatoes, spinach, and red peppers.

Dress it. Let her make her own salad with nutritious greens, such as spinach, kale, arugula, watercress, and romaine. Try an olive oil or canola oil based salad dressing. A tablespoon of hummus stirred into a salad is a healthy alternative to dressing.

Cut it. With a cookie cutter, cut whole wheat bread into fun shapes and make veggie sandwiches.

Grow it. Plant a garden with your child. Help her care for the plants, harvest the veggies, and wash and prepare them. Children are much more likely to eat what they grow. Try a mini-garden on your patio or balcony. If you have birthed several little gardeners, divide their garden into plots and let them name their plants (e.g., "Tommy's tomatoes," "Carol's carrots").

Fill it. Fill veggies with your favorite fillers, such as a stalk of celery filled with lowfat cream cheese, a pocket of whole wheat pita bread filled with hummus and other veggies.

Soy it. When making the switch from meaty to meatless dishes, try tofu in spaghetti sauce instead of meatballs, stir-fried vegetables with tofu cubes, meatless chili (black beans have a meaty texture and some soy subs can pass as meat in chili). Serve soy subs, such as tofu in a stir-fry instead of beef. If switching from beef to veggie burgers (or hot dogs), don't ask and don't tell. Instead of, "How do you like the new kind of burger?" (remember, some kids equate "new" with "yucky") say nothing unless your child detects your trick. Sneak in soy subs to beef whenever you can, such as with sloppy joes (but don't call your sub "sloppy soy!").

Sweeten it. Try zucchini pancakes, carrot cake, pumpkin bread, or bake a pumpkin pie with whole wheat crust.

Friend it. Use peer pressure. Invite over a veggie-loving friend and serve a veggie meal. Create veggie art together.

Lean Choice #2: Eat Smart Proteins

Eating ample protein is an important part of the LEAN Kids Program. Proteins provide the building blocks for growing organs and muscles. Of all the nutrients in food, proteins are the most worry-free. It's hard to eat too much, and you almost never have to worry about children doing so. And, unlike fats and sugars, there is no such thing as an unhealthy protein. As long as it's low in fat, any form of protein is good for your growing child.

PROTEIN PERKS

Proteins have unique features, which make them the darlings of dieters. Each gram of protein contains only four calories, compared with nine calories in a gram of fat. Unlike carbs, proteins don't trigger the roller-coaster effect of the insulin cycle. So eating a lot of protein does not give you the high to low feelings that happen after a rush of junk sugars.

Unlike dietary sugars and fats, excess protein in the diet is not stored as fat. Whatever protein the body doesn't need, it excretes as waste. Proteins are filling without being fattening. Since proteins create a "full and satisfied" feeling quicker than the same grams of carbs, kids are unlikely to overeat high-protein foods the way they do high-sugar stuff. Finally, a high-protein meal or snack usually leaves a person with a more comfortable gut feeling than would be experienced with a high-carb or high-fat meal.

The *minimum* daily requirement that children need from six to twelve years of age is around half a gram per pound of body weight, which translates into a daily protein need of twenty-five to fifty grams, depending on your child's weight. As you will see below, that amount is easy to get in a lean diet. It would be hard to eat more than two grams per pound per day without feeling too full. Children will need to eat more protein during growth spurts, when doing strenuous athletic training, or for tissue repair following an injury or prolonged illness. So, as a general guide, *one gram of protein per pound per day* would be an optimal amount for a child. Remember, if children eat too little protein, they'll make up for it by eating too much fat and carbs.

While we like to see kids on the LEAN Kids Program eat a lot of protein for all these reasons, we want to be clear about the fact that we don't recommend a *protein only* diet. That seems to be the rage for adult dieters these days, and like other diet fads, it just isn't a healthy eating program. Children especially need a fully balanced menu of nutrients, such as the important vitamins and minerals that are available in foods like fruits, vegetables, and whole grains. So while we say, "Eat a lot of protein," we definitely do not advise you to eat *only* protein.

TEACH KIDS ABOUT POWERFUL PROTEINS

Talk about protein foods with your children. Explain the importance of protein for growing muscles, sustained energy, and balanced blood-sugar levels in the body. Also, encourage your children to eat all the protein foods they want.

In fact, because of their biochemical perk of balancing blood-sugar levels, high-protein foods such as yogurt are *the ideal snack foods.* Most packaged snack foods are low in protein, mainly because proteins are more expensive than sugars and fats. Don't expect the food industry to advertise high-protein snacks to your children. Parents have to be the prime protein pushers.

However, once you explain all the benefits of proteins and tell your child they are a free food, you should find him pretty enthusiastic about making the protein lean choice!

The Secret of Salmon

Salmon is one of the top foods on our lean list. It's rich in heart-healthy and brain-building omega-3 oils. Yet not all salmon is created equal. Humans who grow up in a clean environment are healthier than those who grow up in a polluted one, and the same is true with fish. One of the safest and most nutritious foods is wild salmon from the pristine waters of Alaska. Fish farming is illegal in Alaska, and the Alaskan government makes it a high priority to ensure that the water is a clean and nutritious environment for the fish to grow and live. In general, it helps to know where your salmon are raised. We recommend organic meats and organic dairy products for the same reasons that we prefer wild Alaskan salmon.

THE POWERFUL PROTEIN LIST

While all proteins are nutritious, some are more nutritious than others. We've already mentioned that the proteins in lean foods are preferable to those in fatty foods, because animal fats are not good for your heart health. We also recommend organic meats, because we are wary of the antibiotic, hormonal, and steroid additives given to commercially raised beef cattle, chicken, and other animals. We like eating wild game meats in our house, especially bison, which is naturally lean and quite tasty. If you are interested in wild venison, be sure to find out if it is from a region free of the wasting diseases that have infected some of the wild deer in this country. Be sure you buy wild game, since meat from "game farms" may be grain fed and therefore no healthier than beef.

Another way to rank proteins is according to their biological value, which is a measure of how well the body uses the individual amino acid components of a protein. Here's a list of proteins in order of preference according to this measure:

1. Whey protein (human milk)
2. Egg whites
3. Fish
4. Dairy products
5. Beef
6. Soy
7. Legumes

Perhaps the fairest and most practical way of ranking protein foods is to look at the percentage of protein in relation to the total calories in a food, or protein density. For instance, while four ounces of fish and four ounces of lean beef contain equal amounts of protein, *83 percent* of the calories in fish are protein versus only around *40 percent* in beef. So the leanest protein foods usually pack the highest percentage of their calories as proteins. Here's a ranking of foods that pack the most protein as a percentage of the total amount of calories.

We've combined all these different variables into one Powerful Protein list, which are the protein foods we most highly recommend that you and your family focus on in your diet to achieve lean living.

Protein Food	Grams of Protein Per Serving	Protein Density (percentage of calories as protein)
Fish, tuna (4 oz.)	25–30	83%
Egg white (1)	3.5	82%
Cottage cheese, nonfat (½ cup)	15	75%
Poultry, breast, no skin (4 oz.)	25	75%
Salmon (4 oz.)	25	60%
Kidney beans (½ cup)	7	60%
Tofu, firm (3 oz.)	13	45%
Yogurt, plain nonfat (1 cup)	12	40%
Beef, lean (4 oz.)	30	40%
Egg, whole (1)	6	33%
Milk, 1% (8 oz.)	8	32%
Peanut butter (2 tbsp.)	8	17%
Cereal (1 cup) with ½ cup milk	6–8	17%
Nuts or sunflower seeds (1 oz.)	7	16%
Pasta (1 cup)	7	15%
Whole-wheat bread (1 slice)	3	15%

Powerful Proteins

- Fish, especially wild cold-water fish such as salmon and tuna
- Egg, especially egg whites
- Lean meat, especially wild game and organic chicken and beef
- Legumes, especially chickpeas and lentils
- Soy, especially soybeans and tofu
- Nonfat or low-fat organic dairy, especially cottage cheese and yogurt

Lean Choice #3: Eat Smart Carbs

Kids need carbs—lots of them. Carbs give kids the energy they need to play, think, and go! But they need to eat smart carbs. The wrong kind of carbs can cause the worst kind of trouble for your children, unbalancing their hormones to create insulin surges, unhealthy cravings, and the binge eating that follows, all with a minimum of nutrients. On the other hand, the right carbs are crucial in helping your child get through his day with sustained energy, balanced hormones, and adequate vitamins and minerals. More than any other type of food, carbs are a minefield. The wrong carbs are too readily available and the right carbs are too poorly understood. So one of the most important things you need to do in order to live lean is to untangle the confusion about carbs. We'll try to do that for you now.

CARE ABOUT YOUR CARBS

The bottom line is that the best carbs are fiber-filled, and the worst kind aren't. Fiber-filled carbs are digested slowly, and keep your child's blood levels steady. Fiberless carbs are mostly sugar, which the body digests so quickly that your child's blood levels are thrown out of whack. To fully understand the difference between good carbs and bad, let's first understand the lean benefits of fiber.

What's so fantastic about fiber. Fiber has tremendous benefits for kids. It's filling without being fattening, which means it helps curb overeating. High-fiber foods require the child to chew longer. Besides predigesting the food, the prolonged chewing slows down the eating process and allows the child to feel satisfied in time to avoid overeating.

Lean Lesson: Fiber is filling without being fattening.

Fiber-rich foods stay in the stomach longer, absorb water, swell, and help you feel full. Fiber also helps a child move his bowels more regularly and therefore have less bloating and tummy aches.

Because it slows the absorption of sugar from the intestines, fiber (especially the soluble type found in apples, bran, and legumes) steadies the child's blood sugar, lessening the ups and downs of insulin secretion.

Fiber also promotes friendly bacteria. Growing within the intestines of every child and adult are "bad bugs" (those that interfere with intestinal health) and "good bugs" (those that promote intestinal health). Fiber inhibits the growth of harmful bacteria and encourages the growth of beneficial bacteria that aid in the absorption of certain vitamins and essential fats, in addition to lessening the incidence and severity of diarrheal diseases, which children are prone to.

The Age + 5 Fiber Rule

To calculate your child's minimal daily fiber needs, add five grams to your child's age. A nine-year-old would need at least fourteen grams of fiber a day.

What's so bad about sugar. Fiberless carbs are those that have been refined. The kernels of the whole grains have been removed so that the food is easier to digest—too easy! Fiberless carbs come in many forms, especially the sweetened beverages and what I call packaged "bakery bads." As far as your body is concerned, all those fiberless foods are just plain sugar. They enter the bloodstream quickly, induce a surge in insulin and blood-sugar levels, and then cause a burst of energy that is followed by a crash of lethargy and depression. That crash leads to the craving for more food, especially more sugar in some form, which starts the whole cycle again. Also keep in mind that the sweeter the food, the more tempted the child is to *overeat.*

A fast carb is a fat carb. You may have heard someone say, "Sugar is sugar." Not exactly! How sugars behave in your child's body and brain depends upon how quickly they are absorbed into your child's bloodstream. Fiberless carbs (I call them "fast carbs") have a double fault: Because "fast" sugars are absorbed so quickly, the child does not feel full for long and has a tendency to overeat these junk sugars. Secondly, fiberless carbs tend to taste sweeter, and it's easier to overeat sweet foods. These excess fast sugars can then be deposited as excess fat. Remember, fast foods tend to contain more fast sugars.

TEACH YOUR KIDS ABOUT SMART CARBS

Just as it's important for you to understand the difference between fiber-filled and fiberless carbs, your child needs to know how to eat smart carbs. Here are some ways you might explain the truth about carbs to him.

What kids should know about fiber. Most kids understand fiber-rich foods are the ones that take longer to chew—fruits, veggies, and whole grains. Another way to help kids identify good carbs is to explain that they are the fruits, vegetables, and grains that are whole, or closest to their original form.

Some things your kids should know about fiber-rich foods to help them get the most out of them include:

EAT FIBER FOODS FIRST. Eating fiber first helps an overeater feel full and satisfied before he overdoes it.

DRINK LOTS OF WATER WITH FIBER. Fiber acts like an intestinal sponge to soak up water and soften the stools, which allows it to sweep the intestines clean. Without enough water, the fiber can turn into a thick glob that ends up contributing to constipation instead of curing it.

DON'T SKIP THE SKIN. Because the skins of fruits are fiber-rich, we shouldn't peel them. Encourage your child to eat the whole fruit instead of fiberless juice.

THE ABCS OF FAVORITE FIBERS

Most children aren't naturally drawn to high-fiber foods. We've found that once they realize how many of them are also "free foods" (meaning you can eat all you want), the more enthusiastic they get about including them in their diets. Teach your children the following ABCs of fiber foods.

- A: apricots, apples, avocados, artichokes
- B: beans, bran, berries
- C: cereals (those with five grams of fiber per serving)
- S: salads and raw vegetables

Savor Salads

Few children are naturally attracted to salads, which is a shame because they're full of fiber, pack a lot of nutrition into fewer calories, and are plentiful in phytos (nutrients that boost your child's immune system). Here are some tips for making salads a habit for your child:

- Give children salad at the *beginning* of a meal, when they're hungry and less picky about what they eat.
- Include lots of crunches. Many kids dislike salad because they think of it as boring. Toss in chopped carrots, cucumbers, sweet peppers, even raw broccoli or sweet peas—whatever vegetables your child prefers. It will help her develop the salad habit.
- Sprinkle on sunflower seeds instead of croutons.
- Choose great greens. Generally, the darker the greens, the more nutritious the salad. Avoid iceberg lettuce. The best salad greens in nutritional order are spinach, arugula, watercress, endive, and romaine.

- Choose a low-fat, low-calorie dressing and use sparingly, around one tablespoon. A nutritious and tasty alternative to dressing would be a tablespoon or two of hummus mixed into the salad.

Beware of the corn syrup / calorie connection. The natural fructose in fruits and whole foods enjoys a good name among carbs because it doesn't trigger the insulin roller-coaster. Yet this is not true for chemically processed, high-fructose corn syrup (HFCS). This factory-made fructose, the darling of the food industry because it's cheap, may be expensive for the body to metabolize. New studies are showing that it can actually interfere with control of blood sugar, contribute to insulin resistance, and, even more worrisome, raise the level of fats in the blood. I believe the overdrinking of sweetened beverages is the number-one contributor to obesity in children.

Limit Liquid Candy

To remind yourself of exactly what this stuff really is, think of sweetened beverages (especially those corn-syrupy "fruit drinks") as liquid candy. These drinks are mostly syrup or sugar water with a splash of real juice.

What kids should know about sugar. Most school-age children are able to grasp the problem with sugar pretty easily. You just need to explain it in terms they'll understand. For instance, no child likes having a tantrum, especially around friends. It's embarrassing. Ask them to notice how junk sugars make them feel fidgety and giggly at first, but almost always leave them in a bad mood soon afterward. When they have that bad-mood fit two hours after eating cake or candy, remind them that eating sugar is like riding on a roller-coaster. Eating sugary foods like soda, cake, and even pasta is like climbing a hill, and once you reach the top, you have no choice but to plunge down the other side. At the bottom, you feel yucky—and if that's where your child is when you tell the story, the following lesson will sink in.

The Soda Story

One of the worst foods available to our children today are canned, carbonated, sweetened sodas. But they're everywhere and aggressively advertised, so to keep your child off them, you'll have to be pretty persuasive. Try giving them this talk about the anatomy of a soda:

"Kids, here's what happens to your body when you drink a can of soda. You know all that fizzy stuff? What makes it fizzy is a chemical called phosphate. Throughout your body certain chemicals act like partners. You have to have just the right amount of each one so your body works well. Two such partners are calcium and phosphate. When phosphate gets into your bloodstream, it goes looking for its partner, calcium. It steals calcium out of your calcium bank, your bones. Your bones won't grow strong without calcium. Calcium in your bones is like the mortar that keeps bricks together in a building. If the mortar is weak, the brick building will not be strong. So remember, when you drink soda, you weaken your bones.

"And you know that sweet taste you get from pop? Well, can you imagine eating ten teaspoons of sugar all at once? That's exactly what you do when you drink a twelve-ounce can of pop. Some contain even more sugar. When you gulp a big slug of soda, the sugar gets into your body too fast, so your blood-sugar levels go real high and then they crash right down again, and you feel yucky. That yucky feeling is called 'sugar blues,' which is one reason why you might feel so tired in the afternoon after you've had a junk sugar lunch or snack.

"As another insult to the body, sugary drinks cause you to get hungry and overcompensate with increased eating (a metabolic quirk called a high glycemic load). In fact, the more junk sugar you eat, the more junk food you want. You start having cravings you can't control. Also, because fluids are not as filling, calories from fluids can be more fattening than calories from food. It's easier to overdrink than to overeat.

"You know that cute red color? That's also a chemical. It's called a dye. Stick your tongue out after you drink a bright red soda and you'll notice you have a bad case of 'red tongue.' When doctors inject these dyes into rats, some of the rats die of cancer. These dyes are bad for you.

"Kids, let me tell you a secret about what the food industry is doing to you young folks. Because they make a lot of money on you, they flavor the drinks so you want to drink more. They get you in a habit of going to the vending machine and pressing the button on their brand instead of developing a taste for water. I call this shaping young tastes, but the folks who make the soda are shaping your tastes in the wrong direction."

At the same time, you can't really expect children to completely give up sweets. Their sweet-attuned taste buds are actually stronger than those of adults, and it's just natural that kids like sugar. Yet you can try to satisfy their cravings for sweets with more healthful sources than refined sugars. When your child wants something sweet, try giving her one of the substitutes below.

The best carbs are what we call "combo carbs," sugars that are partnered with fiber, fats, and protein. These are also what we call "clean carbs," those that haven't been polluted by processing. Clean combo carbs are smart carbs. They provide a steady release of energy without triggering the highs and lows of blood-sugar swings. And they make great snacks. Because such carbs are more filling and appetite-satisfying

Sweet Subs

- *Cinnamon*: Besides being a sweet spice, cinnamon contains only five calories per teaspoon, yet that includes a gram of fiber, 25 milligrams of calcium, and trace amounts of other vitamins, minerals, and iron. And, as sweet perk, it has a stabilizing effect on blood sugar.

- *Fruit concentrates*: These fructose sugars, besides being sweeter than table sugar and absorbed more slowly, do not trigger the erratic insulin cycle. Because they are sweeter, you can use half as much as table sugar.

- *Fruit toppings*: Used instead of junk syrup, fruit toppings provide some fiber, contain sugars that are absorbed more slowly, and contribute to a more steady blood sugar. Use fresh or frozen blueberries or strawberries, or applesauce.

- *Plain yogurt with fruit*: Fruit sugars are more blood-sugar friendly than corn-syrup sweeteners used in yogurts prepackaged with fruit. If you add the fruit at home, you avoid those junk sugars.

- *Molasses*: One tablespoon contains 172 milligrams of calcium, 3.5 milligrams of iron, and a pinch of many other vitamins and minerals. It is sweeter than table sugar, so you can use half the amount. Blackstrap molasses is the most nutritious kind.

- *A wedge of lemon or lime*: Squirting a bit of lemon or lime juice into plain water will perk up the taste and might show your child that not all drinks have to taste sweet to be good.

- *Fruit juice*: Add one or two ounces of fruit juice to an eight-ounce glass of water to encourage your child to drink more fluids.

than simple carbs, kids are less likely to overeat them. The following are the best combo carbs for kids (and for adults, for that matter).

Smart Combo Carbs

- Fruits
- Legumes (beans, peas, lentils)
- Oatmeal
- Rice (brown or wild)
- Soybeans
- Sweet potatoes
- Veggies
- Whole grains (cereals, pasta, bread)
- Yogurt

Lean Choice #4: Eat Smart Fats

Fat isn't bad for children. In fact, it's necessary for healthy growth. Yet children's needs concerning fats are different from adults'. With the LEAN Kids Program, instead of low-fat eating, we want you adopt "smart-fat" eating. Take a tip from nature (which makes very few nutritional mistakes). Fifty percent of the calories in human milk are supplied by fats. Most school-age children need around *30 percent* of their daily calories in the form of healthy fats. Let's review what you need to know to be a good lean coach for your child on the subject of fats.

SMART FATS

Fat should not be a bad word. We all need some body fat. Without fat we couldn't live, and our bodies wouldn't look very attractive either. Here are ten good things fat does for your body.

1. **Fats build healthy cells.** Picture the cell as a bag of energy. The cell membrane is the bag that holds all the energy in. Since fats form the structural components of the cell membrane, every cell

in the body could fall apart without enough of the right kinds of fats.

2. **Fats build smarter brains.** Fats form the structural components of 60 percent of the brain and nervous system. Besides building better brain cells, fats build myelin, the fatty sheath that insulates the nerves, enabling messages to travel from the brain to other parts of the body.

3. **Fats build healthier skin.** As your child grows, a layer of fat (called subcutaneous fat) forms beneath the skin. This layer of fat regulates body temperature, keeping the child comfortable in hot and cold weather. Too-thin children are more sensitive to the cold; overfat children are more sensitive to hot weather.

4. **Fat helps us look good.** The right amount of body fat, that is. Fat gives our bones and muscles a rounder and more appealing appearance (females naturally have more body fat than males— vive la différence!). You've seen people that look like "just skin and bones." They just don't seem to be filled out in the right places.

5. **Fat protects our insides.** Fat cushions organs, such as the heart, kidneys, and intestines, protecting them from injury.

6. **Fat provides reserve energy.** Children are very active and fat is the body's largest fuel tank, storing energy for the body to use when it needs it.

7. **Fats help vitamins.** The fats in foods help the intestines absorb certain vitamins, such as vitamins A, D, E, and K.

8. **Fats help hormones.** Fats help build important hormones, such as prostaglandin and sex hormones. For example, underweight preteen girls who do not have enough body fat may have delayed puberty. And underweight women of menstruating age can suffer from irregular periods.

9. **Fats build healthy hearts.** What! Fat can be a heart-healthy food? Yes, certain fats can help build a healthy heart. For example, people (such as Eskimos) who eat a lot of fatty seafood rich in omega-3 oils have a lower incidence of heart disease.

10. **Fats help foods taste good.** Eating is supposed to be pleasurable; otherwise the human race wouldn't have survived. Fats give foods a pleasant texture (dubbed "mouth feel" by the food industry). Remember Grandmother's melt-in-your-mouth cookies?

I don't want kids on the LEAN Kids Program to develop a *fat phobia.* Remember, *the wrong kind of fat* is unhealthy, but smart fats are good for you. So in this section we'll show you how to coach your kids to prefer them.

**Lean Lesson: In the LEAN Kids Program,
think right fat, not low fat.**

TEACH KIDS ABOUT RIGHT FATS

Children usually understand the concept of "smart" fats and "dumb" fats. Smart fats are good for your heart and brain. The smartest fats are *omega-3 fats.* These fats are the prime structural components of brain-cell membranes and the insulation coating of the nerves throughout your child's nervous system. Monounsaturated and polyunsaturated fats also help keep your veins free of cholesterol buildup. Consider omega-3s and the mono and poly fats as smart fats. The richest sources of omega-3s, listed in order of food value, are cold-water fish (such as wild salmon and tuna), flax and canola oils, egg yolk, and wild game. There's also a bit in pumpkin seeds and walnuts. Teach your children that the healthiest fats are found in foods that *swim* (fish) or *flow* (oils) and the meat of animals that *run* in the wild. Unhealthy fats are those that just sit there, like the fat on farmed meat and poultry.

Explain to your children that hydrogenated oils are dumb fats. Hydrogenated oils are the ones that are "twisted" so they don't spoil quickly. Explain to your child that she should avoid any food that contains *partially hydrogenated oils* (also known as trans fats). As a general guide, consider foods that contain this to be junk food.

Here are some tips for raising a fat-savvy child:

Shape little fat tastes. Besides being born with a sweet tooth, children have a "fat tooth." Fat helps food taste good. Packaged-food manufacturers call this the "mouth feel" of food. The tastier the mouth feel, the more of the food the child will gobble up. To compete with the mouth feel of junk fats, serve your children good fats so that they get used to the mouth feel of healthy fats. For overfat children who have already been spoiled by the expected fatty tastes of foods, it may take a while to reprogram little taste buds not to expect all food to taste fatty. Yet, after a few months of lean eating, it's likely that the child will crave less fat and actually find the high fat in fast foods distasteful.

Avoid low-fat products. Most packaged-food companies reduce the fat by raising the sugar content of food. Your child is better off eating a smart fat than a low-fat, sugary carb.

Lean Lesson: "Low fat" often means high sugar.

Go fishing! Fish is one of the best foods available, especially because of the fat in it. The earlier you introduce fish into your children's diets, the more likely they will develop a liking for it. The two omega-3 fats (DHA and EPA) found in fish nourish growing brains. The omega-3 fats in fish also nourish the rapidly developing retinas of children's eyes. While fish is one of the top foods for reducing the risk of cardiovascular disease in adults, it also helps keep the blood vessels of little hearts clear of artery-clogging clots—so that your children can avoid developing heart problems. And fish is a rich source of iron, in addition to many vitamins and minerals, a great benefit for children who are prone to iron-deficiency anemia. Besides being a healthy food for growing brains, hearts, and eyes, fish is good for growing muscles. Seafood is one of the most nutrient-dense sources of protein. A four-ounce serving of salmon contains twenty-five grams of protein, the total minimum daily requirement for an average six-year-old. Serve fish two or three times a week as part of the family fare, so that your children grow up learning that "fish is what we eat." Fish, especially wild cold-water fish such as salmon, is a top lean kids food. Remember, studies show that populations who eat the most fish live longer and healthier lives.

Lean Lesson: Fish is good brain food and heart food.

As your child grows, reduce the fat. Infants and toddlers need a higher percentage of their calories as fats than do older children and adults. While infants may need as much as 50 percent of their daily calories as fats, school-age children need no more than *30 percent*, adults no more than 20 percent. I know 30 percent may sound like a lot, but in practice it's not. As your child's coach, you'll need to keep track of how much fat she consumes every day in addition to what kinds of fats.

THE SMART FAT LIST

Try to eat the best fats possible. Here are some suggestions for avoiding or trimming unhealthy fats, and replacing them with smart fats whenever you can.

But of course it's best to stick to the smart fats listed below as often as you can. These are the fats that you should think of as good for you, not bad for you—and try to raise a child who enjoys eating them.

INSTEAD OF . . .	TRY
Whole milk	Low-fat milk
Whole-milk yogurt	Low-fat or nonfat yogurt
High-fat cheeses	Low-fat cheeses
Fatty beef	Lean beef with fat trimmed
Farmed fish	Wild fish
French fries	Sweet potatoes
Dark-meat poultry	White-meat poultry
Beef ("select round" is leaner than "choice" cuts, and "prime" is the fattiest)	Game meats
Beef stir-fry	Tofu stir-fry
Beef burger	Veggie burger
Chicken	Turkey
Sour cream	Low-fat yogurt
Salad dressing	Hummus
Deep-frying	Stir-frying
Frying	Poaching or baking
Frying in oil	Sautéing with chicken broth
Butter on bread	Olive oil on bread

Smart Fats

- Salmon
- Tuna
- Flax oil
- Olive oil
- Canola oil
- Nuts
- Seeds
- Avocado
- Soy foods
- Egg yolk

Lean Choice #5: Water Your Growing Child

Like growing plants, kids need lots of water. Your child's body is 50 to 70 percent water. Getting enough water makes every system of the body work better. As a general guide, your child needs around *an ounce of fluids per pound* of body weight per day, nearly twice as much water per pound of weight than adults, who require around one-half ounce per pound. For example, a fifty-pound six-year-old would need fifty ounces of fluids.

WHAT WATER DOES FOR YOUR CHILD

Children will be more enthusiastic about drinking water if they understand why it's a lean food. As your child's lean coach, you can help him to learn what's so great about water. Here are some reasons to share with your child:

The body's house cleaner. Water keeps the body healthy by helping the kidneys flush toxins out of the body. It's also crucial in helping high-fiber foods sweep your child's bowels clean. Not drinking enough water is the most common cause of constipation in children. The colon is the body's water regulator. If the child doesn't drink enough water, the colon steals it from the stools and gives it to the body.

Water to run. Since muscles are 70 to 75 percent water, when children are even slightly dehydrated, they get tired and don't perform as well. Also, water lubricates those growing little joints that need to move so fast.

Drink Before You're Thirsty

Encourage your children to drink water *before* they become thirsty. Thirst is not a reliable indication of water need, since by the time you feel thirsty, your body is already depleted by at least two cups of water.

Water to think. Like muscles, the brain is 70 to 75 percent water. So, when it's water deprived, it doesn't think right. Teach your child, "Drink to think." Hydration improves concentration. Headaches can be caused by dehydration.

Water to breathe. When a child has a cold, especially with a fever, he breathes faster and perspires more, which causes the body to lose water. This may cause the membranes of the breathing passages to dry out and get plugged with thick mucus. Waterlogging the mucous membranes keeps the secretions caused by a cold from plugging up the airways. Water is the best and least expensive "cough syrup."

Water to not itch. The skin loves water. If it doesn't get enough of it, it dries out and gets itchy and flaky. If you notice your child scratching frequently, she needs more water.

Water controls overeating. Some overweight kids eat too much, but drink too little. If your child is a compulsive overeater, invite her to drink a glass of warm water before every meal. That water can curb the appetite and dampen the urge to overeat.

Water helps weight loss. Here's a drinking deal you can't resist! Drinking extra water helps you lose excess fat. When cool water reaches warm intestines, your body must burn calories to produce heat to bring the water up to body temperature. Here's the math. If you give your child an extra quart of cold water a day, the body would burn enough extra calories to lose two to three pounds of fat per year.

Beware of the Water Robbers

Certain drinks can steal water from your child's body rather than replenish it. Caffeine-containing drinks have a diuretic effect, meaning they cause the kidneys to excrete water. Let's follow two drinks through the intestines so you can see how plain water hydrates better than junk drinks. When the child drinks plain water, most of the water is rapidly absorbed through the intestines into the bloodstream and circulates throughout the body to where it is needed. Any excess is urinated out. Now add a bunch of caffeine, sugar, and corn syrup to the water. These additives lessen the amount of water that is absorbed by the intestines. Large doses of caffeinated, high-sugared juices can even produce diarrhea, which increases the water loss from the intestines. The main lean message to give your children: *When thirsty, drink water.*

TIPS FOR WATERING KIDS

Most kids like water, especially if you introduce them to it as infants and make it a regular part of their diet every day. But not all kids do. Here are some ways to make water part of your child's life.

"Water is what we drink." Model for your children that water is the family drink. Let them see you drinking lots of water. Continually surround your child with the message that "water is what we mainly drink. Other drinks are an occasional treat." Like veggies are a "free food" in lean eating, tell your children that "water is a free drink. Drink as much as you want."

"We don't drink junk juice." Contradict the ads for junk juice and soft drinks that your child is constantly bombarded with on television.

Anytime you see a junk beverage ad, talk about how much healthier plain water is.

Water, water everywhere. Plant water bottles within easy reach throughout the house. Put water bottles by everyone's bedside. Serve water at mealtimes. Put a small bottle of water in your child's backpack. Keep water in the car. Make a water bottle your child's constant companion.

Drink Waterade Instead of Sports Drinks

Except when your child is exercising strenuously for more than an hour, water is a better (or equally effective) hydrator than sports drinks. A sports drink may contain a lot of extra sugar, colorings, and chemicals that shape young tastes toward craving these flavors. Sports drinks also have a lot of salt, which help rehydrate the body after strenuous exercise, but that benefit comes at the cost of a lot of added junk food. A child will do better with a bottle of water and a bit of fruit before a game rather than a junky sports drink. Or, you can make your own carbo-drink for your child to have during strenuous exercise. A teaspoon of salt and a pinch of cinnamon added to a quart of 100 percent, noncarbonated juice is a nutritious sports drink.

Shape young tastes toward water. If your child resists plain water, flavor it by adding the juice from a wedge of lemon, lime, or orange. Or add an ounce of 100 percent juice to increase flavor.

Serve water-rich foods. If your child remains reluctant to drink water, serve waterlogged foods such as watermelon, soups, and fruit-rich smoothies. These foods are 80 to 90 percent water.

Traffic-Light Eating

There's a lot to remember when becoming a lean eater. If much of this information is new to you, it might feel a little overwhelming. Rest assured that as you live the LEAN Kids Program, these healthy choices will become second nature to you.

I have found that people new to the program find it useful to have an easy reminder of what foods to emphasize and which to avoid. Working with lean kids in our practice, we found that some kids enjoy making healthy food choices by relating them to traffic lights.

"Green light" foods are "go for it" foods; they're great for you. "Yellow light" foods are "think about it" foods; they're okay in moderation but should be reserved to accompany a meal of primarily green-light foods. "Red light" foods are to stop; try to avoid them.

Tape the following chart to your refrigerator so your family can see which foods can be eaten frequently (green light), which foods can be eaten in moderation (yellow light), and which foods to avoid (red light).

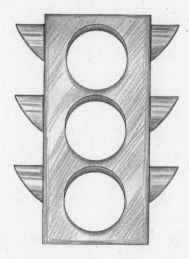

TRAFFIC LIGHT LIST

Green-Light Foods	Yellow-Light Foods	Red-Light Foods
Enjoy; go for it	Slow down; enjoy, but not too much	Stop and think about a healthier choice
• All fruits • All veggies • Cheese, low-fat • Eggs • Flaxseed oil • Meat, lean • Milk, low-fat • Nuts and seeds • Olive oil • Salmon • Soy foods, e.g. tofu • Whole grains • Yogurt	• Butter • Cookies, homemade • Frozen yogurt • Fruit juice, 100 percent • Honey • Meats, fatty • Pasta • Pastries, homemade • White bread	• Beverages, presweetened with sugar or corn syrup • Cottonseed oil • Dyes • Foods with artificial sweeteners • Foods with hydrogenated oils • Prepackaged or store-bought bakery goods • Gelatin desserts • Marshmallows • Nitrite-containing meats

The Grow Food Plate

In the past couple of years, we've seen the government-sponsored nutritional pyramid come under fire, mainly because it does not differentiate between whole foods and processed ones. As the exact nature of the healthiest diet is debated more and more, that pyramid gets more and more confusing. For the Lean Kids Program we've formulated a guideline that we call the Grow Food Plate. The goal of our nutritional plate is the same as the government's nutritional pyramid: It's an easy visual way of remembering how much to eat of different kinds of foods.

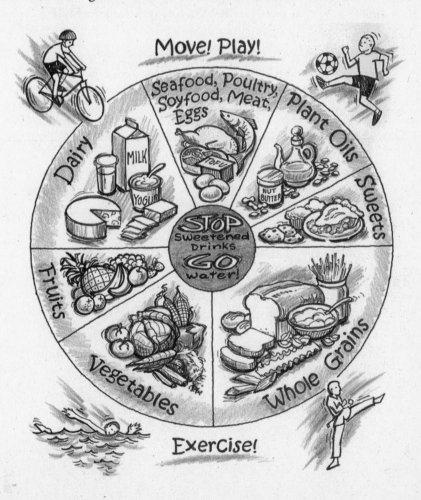

Guide to the Grow Food Plate

Keep in mind:

- Our guide is based on an average 2,000-calorie-per-day diet, the average amount for a ten-year-old. This amount will vary from day to day depending on the child's activity level. (Becoming calorie conscious is discussed in the next chapter.)
- The nutritional breakdown is:
  Carbs (50–55% of daily calories) are fiber-filled and nutritious.
  Fats (25–30% of daily calories) are mostly from heart-healthy seafood and plant sources.
  Protein makes up 15–20% of the total daily calories.
- The plate is based primarily on whole foods and in proportions that promote growth and health.

Foods and serving size explanations:

- **Dairy:** yogurt, milk, low-fat cheese, 3 servings daily (300–400 calories)
  Serving size: 1 cup of milk or yogurt, ½ cup cottage cheese, ½ ounce cheese
- **Seafood, soy food, lean meat, poultry:** 3 times a week (200 calories)
  Serving size: 4 ounces
- **Plant oils:** nut butters, nuts, flaxseed oil, olive oil, 2 tablespoons daily (200 calories)
  Serving size: 1 ounce nuts and seeds, 2 tablespoons nut butter
- **Eggs:** 1 egg, 5 times a week (75 calories)
- **Sweet treats:** baked goods, homemade with whole grains and plant-oil fats and fruit-concentrate sugars, 3 to 5 times a week (100–200 calories)

10

NUTRITION

How to Eat

Now that you know what to eat on the LEAN Kids Program, it's time to talk about *how* to eat. You may think your child knows how to eat all too well, but the truth is that in today's modern society nothing could be further from the truth. In fact, most of us (even our young children) have lost some or all of our original Wisdom of the Body that guided us naturally to eat in a healthful way. Because of that, I have found most kids starting the LEAN Kids Program need some practical guidelines for re-learning how, when, and where to eat (as well as the "what" we covered in chapter 9). It might be interesting as you review this chapter to ask your child to tell you how much of this he already knows. How much do you know?

Children Don't Need to Count Calories

We've said this before but we'll say it again, because it's so important: We do not advocate calorie counting for children for a lot of reasons.

First, it's too hard for most six-to-twelve-year-olds to keep track of calorie consumption throughout the day. They won't count calories themselves, and they probably also will not be able to keep an accurate record of what they eat so that you can count calories for them.

Second, I find that calorie counting can lead to unhealthy attitudes toward food. We want children to understand that *it's not always how much they eat that matters, it's what they eat that makes them fat or lean.* If they are making the wise food choices discussed throughout this chapter, they will seldom need to worry about how many calories to eat.

LOOKING AT PORTION SIZE

Yet, having said all that, we also know that if you have an overfat child who has forgotten how to stop eating when she's full, you (as her lean coach) probably want calorie guidelines to help her learn appropriate portion sizing. We'll provide those guidelines for you here, but you must be careful to use them only as a general guide to portion sizing. Don't get too rigid about these amounts, or you'll do your child more harm than good.

Most children from six to twelve years of age need from 1,500 to 2,000 calories a day (around 30 calories per pound of optimal body weight per day), divided into roughly 20 percent protein, 50 percent nutritious carbs, and 30 percent healthy fats. Yet, there is a wide range of caloric requirements, depending on a child's basic metabolism and activity level. Children naturally need more during heavy exercise (approximately 300 extra calories per hour of strenuous exercise). Assuming a sedentary child, the calorie requirements could break down for each meal as follows in the chart below. (More active children need to eat more.)

If you want to work with these guidelines in mind, we recommend that you get a calorie guide and consult it when planning your child's meals. But don't let your child see what you're doing. And, as you learn the basic caloric values of different foods, put the book away. It won't take you long to re-educate yourself about appropriate portion sizes, and the sooner you can depend on your common sense, the better.

BIG AND SMALL EATERS

What if you have two children, one who is a big eater and one who is a picky eater? How can you keep one from getting too fat and the other from being undernourished?

By understanding the basic nutritional principles called *caloric density* (CD)—the number of calories in a certain weight or volume of a serving of food—and *nutrient density* (nutrients per calorie), you can use these principles to optimally feed children with both of these eating patterns.

MEAL	AVERAGE CALORIES
Breakfast	500
Snack	200
Lunch	500
Snack	200
Dinner	500
Snack	100
Total for Day	**2000**

For the child who seems to eat too much (alias "the big eater"), celebrate that he likes to eat. Don't try to change how much he eats, but nutritionally monitor what he eats, which is the principle of lean eating anyway. To enjoy eating, this child needs to see big portions. His grandmother would say, "His eyes are bigger than his stomach." In this case, to satisfy both his eyes and his stomach, feed him foods with a low calorie density. These are foods with a high water and fiber content, which look like big portions but have fewer calories. These foods are mainly fruits and vegetables. Try the three S's: salads, soups, and smoothies. Begin the meal with low-CD foods, such as soup and salad. Then, as the meal progresses, increase the calorie density of the food. Because this child is satisfied with the big portions at the beginning of the meal, he's unlikely to overeat by the time the meal is over. I was a big eater as a child. Perhaps that's why my grandmother put a big grapefruit (only eighty calories) in my school lunch bag.

For the child who seems to eat too little, try the reverse strategy: Emphasize foods with a high calorie density. These are foods that pack a lot of nutrition in a smaller volume. This child would do better beginning the meal with an entrée, such as a salmon fillet or a patty of lean beef, and saving the salad for after the meal.

Examples of low-CD foods are nearly all vegetables and most fruits. Examples of high-CD foods are meat, seafood, avocados, nuts, and nut butters. Serve the big eater a cupful of *grapes* (low CD) and the small eater a handful (¼ cup) of *raisins* (high CD). Both contain the same number of calories and similar nutrition, yet their different sizes appeal to different appetites.

Keep in mind that caloric density applies only to whole foods from nature, such as fruits, vegetables, grains, seafood, and meat. It does not apply to processed foods. Obviously, a glass of skim milk and a glass of cola could contain the same number of calories in the same volume, yet one is nutritious and one is not. This is why the concept of *nutrient density* (nutrients per calorie) is important in lean eating. Lean foods (such as milk and yogurt) tend to have high nutrient densities, yet processed foods (like sweetened beverages) tend to have low nutrient densities. Ideally, you want to feed your children nutrient-dense foods as much as possible, regardless of their weight.

ENJOY FREE FOODS

The best way to get over a dependence on calorie counting is to embrace the concept of free foods. What are free foods? These are foods that even if eaten in large amounts are unlikely to make your child overfat, for several reasons. First, these foods tend to be high in fiber and quickly filling, so the child is unlikely to overeat. Second, by a lean little biochemical quirk, the body uses almost as many calories to chew and digest vegetables as there are in the veggies in the first place. Third, many of these foods have a high water content (e.g., fruits and veggies), so your child can eat big portions without getting a big belly.

These three facts combine to describe foods that your child can enjoy while they naturally train her not to overeat, because they're so filling. While the idea of a "free food" is that your child can eat as much as he likes, the quirk of free foods is that they are so filling and satisfying that they remind your child of what a sensible portion size is according to his "tummy feel" rather than a scale or calorie-counting book.

The free food list tends to be longer for children than it is for adults, because kids burn more calories per pound of body weight than adults do. Remember: *Children rarely get overfat from overeating lean foods.*

FREE FOODS

- All vegetables
- All fruits
- All lean meat and fish, and especially salmon
- Eggs
- Green, leafy vegetables
- Legumes (beans, peas, lentils)
- Soy foods (soybeans, tofu)
- Whole grains

Begin the Day with a Brainy Breakfast

Mom was right—breakfast is the most important meal of the day. Many kids don't have an appetite for food when they first wake up, and many of us are in such a rush to get our families up and out for the day that we don't have time for breakfast either. Yet once you understand everything breakfast can do for your child, you'll never skip it again.

BREAKFAST BENEFITS

Eating breakfast perks up the metabolism, which perks up the brain. Research has shown that when compared with their breakfast-skipping peers, breakfast eaters are more likely to achieve higher grades, pay closer attention, participate more in class discussions, and manage more complex academic problems. Breakfast primes the brain for learning.

Breakfast skippers tend to be more overfat than breakfast eaters. Breakfast sets the nutritional tone for the day. When children eat a good breakfast, they are more likely to eat lean the rest of the day. When children miss breakfast, they get overly hungry and tend to overeat at lunch time. Also, research has shown that kids who eat a high-sugar breakfast tend to overeat junk food the rest of the day.

School Breakfasts Build Smarter Kids

Research on the National School Breakfast Program showed that compared with children who rarely ate breakfast, those who began the day with a nutritious school breakfast:

- Averaged math scores a whole letter grade higher.
- Showed less tardiness and missed fewer school days because of illness.
- Improved their reading scores.
- Suffered less depression, anxiety, and hyperactivity.
- Were more attentive.
- Showed improved memory on complex tasks.

WHAT MAKES FOR A BRAINY BREAKFAST?

What does the LEAN Kids Program consider a good breakfast? Here's a clue: It doesn't come in a brightly colored box and sugar is not the primary ingredient! Instead, a balanced brainy breakfast has lots of protein, complex carbohydrates, and fiber, as well as calcium and some fats. Proteins perk up the brain and complex carbohydrates relax the brain, so the right balance of both stimulate and relax the brain for optimal performance. Fiber steadies the absorption of the nutrients, so they act like a time-release energy capsule throughout the morning and prevent midmorning crashes and sugar cravings. High-calcium foods have been shown to enhance behavior and learning in schoolchildren. A bit of fat (primarily omega-3s) also steadies the absorption of food and enhances brain performance.

The Science of a Brainy Breakfast

The USDA wanted to know why kids who ate a good breakfast did so much better in school, so they sponsored a symposium on breakfast and learning in children in Washington, D.C., on April 22, 1999. The experts concluded that a brainy breakfast helps a child's brain utilize glucose better. While the brain makes up only 2 percent of the weight of the body, it uses about 25 percent of the body's blood sugar. The physiologic basis for the brainy breakfast/better performance correlation seems to be that when breakfast skippers try to perform complex learning tasks, the brain runs out of fuel because it depletes the marginal glucose stores from the overnight fast. The brain of a child who refuels before school does not run out of glucose while performing complex learning tasks. Simply put, breakfast skippers run out of gas; breakfast eaters have lots of fuel reserves that are not depleted by complex learning.

BUILDING A BRAINY BREAKFAST

The best way to get your kids hooked on breakfast is to make it a meal that's fun and leaves them feeling great. Here are some suggestions for creating your personal best breakfast.

Keep a food-mood diary. Some children are more sensitive than others in terms of the influence of food on their behavior and learning. Keep a journal listing which foods perk up your child and which foods let him down. Let your child help you construct the diary; encourage him to tell you about his school day. Before too long you'll begin to see a pattern in what he has for breakfast on a good day and what he has on a bad day. He'll notice, too!

Keep calm. Not only does the food that your child eats at the beginning of the day affect learning and behavior, so does the family mood. Breakfast time, or the before-school hour, is not the time to get into family arguments or stress your child. There's a biochemical reason for this.

Stress hormones, in addition to affecting behavior, increase the cravings for sugary foods. You don't want your child to be craving doughnuts as soon as he gets to school. Make your child's breakfast a "happy meal."

LEAN KIDS SAY

"The morning is a good time. Either my mom or my dad will make a smoothie with all kinds of good stuff. The smoothies make me feel good and they're sweet and also a whole lot better than just juice."
—JACOB, AGE NINE

Be open to the weird. While we are used to thinking of a nutritious breakfast as a combination of grains, fruit, and dairy, any combo of proteins, complex carbs, and healthy fats is all right. After all, the Japanese enjoy fish for breakfast. (Seafood, rich in omega-3 fats and proteins, actually tops the list of brain foods.) If your child wants pizza (nutritious ingredients, please!) for breakfast, celebrate her different cuisine.

Drink and drive. Some kids resist breakfast just because of the time it takes, especially late sleepers. These children can often be convinced to join the breakfast crowd if you can give them the meal to go. In our house, we've found the easiest way to do that is to make a nutrient-packed smoothie. You'll find our favorite recipe below (see Dr. Bill's Schoolade on page 206), but you can always design your own.

TEN BRAINY BREAKFAST SUGGESTIONS

Still not sure what to serve? If years of brightly colored, sugary cereals have dulled your creative senses, you'll appreciate the list below. These brainy breakfast suggestions should appeal to most kids.

1. Scrambled eggs, whole-wheat toast, and calcium-fortified orange juice

2. High-fiber, high-protein cereal with low-fat milk and fresh fruit
3. Peanut butter and banana slices on a whole-wheat English muffin, with low-fat milk
4. Veggie omelet with whole-wheat toast and a glass of low-fat milk
5. Whole-grain pancakes or waffles topped with berries and yogurt, and a glass of calcium-fortified orange juice
6. Low-fat cheese melted on toast, and a piece of fruit
7. Low-fat cheese, tomato sauce, and veggies on a whole-grain pizza crust, and a glass of low-fat milk
8. Two soft-boiled eggs, stewed tomatoes, a slice of lean ham, and whole-wheat toast
9. Low-fat cream cheese and smoked fish on a whole-grain bagel, with orange juice
10. Dr. Bill's Schoolade recipe

THE SIPPING SOLUTION

This lean way of eating is a liquid version of grazing. In our medical practice, we've successfully used this technique, especially for very obese children and adults who need to downsize their appetites. I discovered this sipping solution, and the Schoolade recipe, in order to jump-start my own personal LEAN Program six years ago. I felt so good and had so much energy that I have continued this way of eating most days of the week ever since. Drinking and sipping is a good way to initially reprogram your body to enjoy the lean way of eating. Here's how it's done: Enjoy two cups of Schoolade as a quick breakfast and then put the remaining amount in a large container that you can keep in a cooler or refrigerator. Every couple of hours throughout the day, give it a vigorous shake and sip. Sipping throughout the day keeps your blood sugar steady and gets you used to feeling satisfied—not uncomfortably full and not hungry. Try this for a couple of weeks as you begin the LEAN Program.

Dr. Bill's Schoolade

Here's the recipe for everyone's favorite smoothie in the Sears house.

3 cups low-fat milk or soy beverage

1½ cups yogurt

1 banana

1 tsp. lemon juice (to preserve color)

1 cup frozen blueberries

½ cup of several of your favorite frozen fruits (e.g., mango, pineapple, organic strawberries)

4 tbsp. ground flaxseeds (for a grainy texture) or 2 tbsp. flaxseed oil (for a silky texture)

4 ounces tofu

2 tbsp. peanut butter

¼ cup raisins (optional)

2 tbsp. wheat germ (optional)

cinnamon and nutmeg to taste

2 servings of a chocolate- or vanilla-flavored multinutrient supplement (optional; see www.leankids.com/schoolade for recommendations)

Serving suggestions: Combine all the ingredients, blend until smooth, serve immediately when it has a bubbly, milkshake consistency.

Nutritional breakdown: One average serving size for a child aged six to twelve would be 2½ cups (20 ounces). One serving would provide a perfect nutritional balance for a brainy breakfast: 500 calories, 8 grams of fiber, and 25 grams of protein; 30 percent fat (mostly healthy omega-3s and monounsaturated fats), 20 percent protein, and 50 percent complex carbohydrates. This recipe makes around eight cups, just right for three school-age children or a family of three.

Lean Perk: Breakfast Moves Little Bowels

Constipation is a common problem in school-age children (especially boys) who may be too busy to listen to their bowel signals or too embarrassed to ask to go to the bathroom. High-fiber, high-fluid natural laxatives (especially the fruit and flax in the smoothie recipe above) and intestines-friendly yogurt all add up to move those little bowels when they should. It helps school children to begin their day with a morning movement.

Lean Habits at Mealtime

Lean is not just a question of what you eat, but how you eat it. In other words, the way you behave at mealtimes can be crucial to your overall health. And we're not talking about keeping your elbows off the table and your napkin in your lap (although those things are nice, too). The following lean-eating tips will help your children get the most nutrition—and the most satisfaction—out of each bite. As a result of these practical bite-by-bite suggestions, your children will not only become leaner, but they will actually get more pleasure from their meals.

DOWNSIZE YOUR CHILD'S SERVINGS

Super-sized foods and drinks like Big Macs, Big Gulps, Double-doubles, and Whoppers have created big waists. They are advertised as better values, but the truth is that they do more harm than good. And the problem is that our children are especially vulnerable to this kind of advertising. Children tend to think that they can eat more than their tummies can hold. You've heard that children's eyes are bigger than their stomachs. There is some truth to this saying. The fact is that a child's stomach is about the size of her fist. So, obviously, a super-sized *anything* is too big a portion for her.

Does overeating stretch the stomach? Animal studies have shown that gorgers quickly develop larger stomachs, allowing and encouraging them to eat more. After all, the stomach is mostly a big bag of muscle. If you stretch it, it's going to get bigger. If an overeater grows up with an over-stretched stomach, it's possible that his appestat (the gauge in his brain that registers when he is full) could be reset *higher,* so he needs to eat more to feel satisfied.

In our medical practice, I have noticed that after several months of lean eating, both adults and children report that they *feel satisfied with less food* and feel uncomfortable consuming the big portions they used to eat. So as you and your family get started on the LEAN Kids Program, always encourage small portions. Don't serve them on adult-size plates, because that suggests that you expect your children to eat adult-size portions. By presenting smaller portions on smaller plates, you send the message that you expect them to eat a child's portion. If they complain, remind them that they can always ask for more. Be sure to wait until at least twenty minutes after your meal has started before serving seconds, and check with your child to see if she still wants more. That will give her body time to know if it's really full or not.

If the idea of downsizing servings is completely new to you, here are a few tricks you can use to get started.

- Let your child serve herself. While some children have eyes that are bigger than their tummies, on the whole studies show that kids tend to select smaller or more appropriate-sized portions than the ones their parents serve them.
- Avoid asking your child, "Would you like more?" If he's hungry enough, he'll ask!
- Never, ever tell your child to "clean your plate." Your child should base his decision about when to stop eating on the feeling in the tummy, not on the appearance of his plate. If you hate the idea of wasting food, wrap it up and save it for later. But don't force it on your child.

- Don't put bowls of food on the dinner table. Fill each plate with an appropriate serving and leave the bowls on the kitchen counter. Out of sight is often out of mind, and out of tummy.
- Give the overeater an apple just before dinner; the fiber and pectin in the apple will help keep him from eating too much at dinner.

TAKE SMALL BITES

Along with smaller portions, children also learn to take smaller bites. Smaller bites give the taste buds a chance to *savor the flavor* of the food, in addition to making chewing and digestion easier. Big bites force most food past the tongue too quickly for flavor to be absorbed. In addition, if you can't taste it, why eat it? Small bites also help make the meal last longer, which gives your stomach enough time to signal to your brain that you're full—so that you don't overeat.

Yet, as sensible as small bites are, the truth is that children (especially between the ages of six and twelve) sometimes just *love* to stuff the food in their mouth. Sometimes it's because they are impatient to get the mealtime over with. Sometimes it's because it's just a game. Whatever the reason, it can be hard to get them to reverse their behavior.

Here are some suggestions for slowing down your speedy eater:

- Cut your child's food into small bites.
- Give her a small fork.
- Play a game with your child to see how small her bites can be.
- Serve her an age-appropriate portion and then ask her if she can make twenty bites (or whatever number makes sense with what you're eating) out of it.

PLAY CHEW-CHEW

Getting your children to thoroughly chew their food can sometimes be even harder than getting them to take small bites. Mom's mealtime sermons to "chew your food thoroughly" was biochemically sound and will help keep your child lean. The longer food lingers in your mouth, the easier it is to digest. Chewing breaks up the fiber that holds the food together, like unwrapping a food package. It gives digestive enzymes easier access to work on the food inside. Chewing stimulates saliva, which not only lubricates the upper digestive tract for smoother passage and comfortable eating, but also protects it against the irritating effects of stomach acids. Saliva is the body's own health juice. Saliva is rich in enzymes that predigest the food, saving work—and rumbling—in your stomach and intestines.

So, how do you get your child to slow down and chew more? Here are some ideas:

- Count chews. Encourage your child to chew each bite at least ten to twenty times. You might even offer a reward to your child if he can chew every bite in a meal that many times.
- Encourage your child to explore the textures of food. Ask her, "How many chews does it take to chew your steak thoroughly?" Compare that to "How many times do you have to chew your

When Do We Stop Listening to Our Tummies?

In a 2000 study, Penn State researchers looked at the effect of increasing food portions on two age groups of children. They presented three-year-olds with increasing serving sizes, yet these children didn't succumb to super-sizing. They stopped eating when full and left the unwanted food on their plates. Not so the five-year-olds, who kept right on eating. From this study we can conclude that once kids reach middle childhood (ages six to twelve), their eating cues become less self-controlled and require more parental guidance. In other words, if you're reading this book, you will probably have to make a conscious effort to re-educate your child—and yourself—about what "enough" is at mealtime.

mashed potatoes?" This, too, will seem like a game to your child, and she might even enjoy putting the results of each bite into a chart.

EAT SLOWLY

The goal behind small bites and thorough chewing is really to help teach your child to eat slowly. Eating slowly is crucial to lean eating because it gives your child's stomach time to signal the brain that it's full before your child overeats. Eating slowly is the most natural and effective form of portion control.

There is a mechanism in the hypothalamus of the brain dubbed the *appestat*, which controls your appetite. The appestat is designed to register when you are satisfied and cue you to stop eating. There is a delay of approximately *twenty minutes* between the time the food fills the tummy and the appestat registers "enough!" This is why slowing down the pace at which you consume your food is so important.

Encouraging your child to take small bites and chew well are the first steps. Here are some other ideas about how to help your child take more time to dine:

- Ask your child to put down her fork after every few bites.
- Encourage your child to take a drink after every few bites.
- Stop and take a few deep breaths between bites with your child.
- Show your child how to use a napkin between bites.
- After every bite, ask your child a question about her day.
- Play Twenty Questions with your child, but only allow him to ask questions between bites.

Don't forget to always allow a naturally slow eater to take his time. Sometimes, parents themselves are in such a rush to get dinner served, eaten, and cleaned up that they feel impatient with a child who dawdles over his meal. Yet the truth is that those procrastinators are eating the right way, and the rest of the family should try to match their pace!

TALK TO YOUR TUMMY

Tell your child that when her tummy fills full, stop eating. Sounds simple, but far too few Americans pay attention to their body's built-in portion monitor. Usually, kids overeat because they're not paying attention to how their tummy feels (unlike adults, who often overeat for emotional reasons). When your body realizes you've eaten enough, it sends a message (the satiety signal) to your brain's neurotransmitters (especially serotonin) to say, "Enough already, you're satisfied. Stop eating." For the compulsive overeater, stop mid-meal and ask your child, "Are you full yet?" That will help him learn to always ask himself. And if you've succeeded in getting your child to slow down, take small bites, and chew her food, chances are that more than twenty minutes will have passed when you ask her if she's full—and she'll say, "Yes!"

ENJOY HAPPY MEALS

A true "happy meal" doesn't come with a toy. A real happy meal is a relaxed family dinner. The happier and more relaxed you are while dining, the less likely you are to overeat mindlessly. The more relaxed you are, the more saliva you produce. This gives a head start on digestion and leads to a more comfortable gut feeling. Keep this in mind when enjoying family dinners. Keeping the conversation happy at mealtimes gives your family a better chance of eating less and enjoying it more.

Not only does eating at home improve family eating habits and help the family get lean, but it can make the whole family happier, too. Research shows that families who frequently eat dinner together have children who have a better sense of values, show improved school performance, and engage in less risky behavior.

Lean Habits Throughout the Day

Lean eating is not just a question of what you eat or your mealtime behavior. Lean eating is something you do all day. Lean eating defines your relationship with food on every level. And if your child has a weight problem, it probably means she has a lot of habits to release. Here are some important habits to teach your children to help them stay lean all the time.

EAT MINDFULLY

As part of binge-proofing, teach your child to keep her mind on what she's eating. Mindless eating sets up a child for overeating. Don't let kids eat while they're watching TV, reading, talking on the phone, or engaging in any other activity besides conversation.

Most kids have a lot of trouble not eating while they watch TV. That's because sitting for prolonged periods of time is unnatural for children. They're fidgety because they're bursting with energy! The exercise program we discussed in chapter 7 will help cut down on TV snacking by giving them something healthful to do with all those fidgets. You might also suggest that your child try engaging in some of the following activities while he watches TV: drawing, sewing, knitting, building (with blocks, Legos, or train sets), or board games.

Explain that meals in your home are eaten at the kitchen or dining room table. Discuss why there is such a danger of overeating if you indulge in food in the midst of another activity or quickly grab a handful of something while you're standing at the kitchen counter. Your child

---

Uncouple Your Child

Couplings, or food associations, trigger cravings, because in the child's brain a pattern of association between TV watching and chip munching has been formed. Try a technique dubbed "uncoupling" to break the common food-TV combo. My advice is to make a rule that in your family, "we don't eat in the TV room." Tell your child that if she wants something to eat (especially if it's the kind of unhealthful snack she used to gobble down while watching her favorite shows), she has to eat it in the kitchen. Your rule will cut down on mindless eating.

should understand that *her food deserves her attention*, and she will enjoy it more if she makes a conscious activity out of eating it.

AVOID BOREDOM EATING

Second only to the mindless eating children do in front of the TV is their turning to food when they have nothing else to do. Children often turn to the refrigerator for satisfaction when what they are really craving is something to do and someone to do it with. When you see your children moving around the kitchen, take some time to help them find another activity. Or, better yet, take a break to play with them yourself. Keep your child busy so that she can keep her mind off food between meal and snack times.

While you want your children to eat mindfully at mealtimes, you don't want them to be thinking about food all the time. If you think about food, your stomach imagines it's going to soon get fed and begins preparing itself by secreting stomach acids. These acids want something to digest, so you eat. The more you get your mind off of food *between meals*, the more your stomach will oblige.

DON'T GO HUNGRY

Remember that the goal of lean eating is to teach children to listen to their body's cues, so they gain control over their eating habits. While your child should avoid thinking about food all the time, she should think about food when she's hungry. The hunger cue is very strong and should be heeded right away. The longer you ignore it, the stronger it gets—which sets you up for bingeing and overeating to catch up. Hunger also lowers the resting metabolic rate, which is the last thing you want in an already sedentary child.

A parent once asked me, "How do you know when a child is hungry?" To answer this question, let's take a look at the difference between hunger and appetite. Hunger, by definition, is a physiological *need* for food (meaning energy). Appetite, on the other hand, is a psychological *desire* for food. Our bodies give us early signs ("hunger pangs") that we need food. If we don't listen to these signals and eat we feel weak, tired, cranky, or shaky, or get headaches. Should you allow your body to get to a point when you experience these sensations? The answer is obviously no.

One of the most important things the LEAN Kids Program has to teach you and your child about lean eating is that you should eat when you're hungry, make it a mini-meal, consume it mindfully and with full enjoyment—and then don't think about food again until you get your next hunger pang!

ENCOURAGE GOOD GRAZING

The best way to avoid hunger is to graze. Tiny children have tiny tummies, about the size of their fists. Encourage your child to graze on frequent, nutritious mini-meals (as many as five to seven, or every two to three hours) throughout the day, rather than three big meals. Kids who eat small, frequent, *nutritious* meals throughout the day tend to have less excess body fat than those who eat two or three large meals.

Here's some recent research that shows how great grazing is.

- Students who ate a 200- to 300-calorie snack fifteen minutes before a test scored 15 to 20 percent higher than those who ate nothing before the test.
- Grazers tend to have lower blood levels of insulin, total cholesterol, and LDL (bad cholesterol), all indicators of health risks.
- Animals who consume their whole day's rations at one time become fatter than animals that eat mini-meals every few hours, even when the total daily caloric consumption is the same for both. Animal studies have shown that gorgers quickly develop larger stomachs, allowing them to eat more.
- People on grazing diets sometimes eat more calories than gorgers eat, but in these studies, the gorgers still wound up fatter.

Here's what happens when you gorge rather than graze. Gorging on a big meal causes a dramatic rise in blood insulin levels, followed by a dramatic drop. Just like too much sugar, huge meals cause the child to initially feel lethargic and then soon crave more food.

Grazing, on the other hand, is an *eat-as-you-burn* way of lean eating. Grazing on lean foods throughout the day promotes steady blood insulin levels. When this master hormone is steady, all the other hormones in the body tend to be steady.

Be careful not to mistake grazing for thinking about and eating food constantly. The secret to grazing is to keep the meals tiny (snacks, really), to stop eating when you're full, and to not think about food again until you feel hungry. The truth is, this is the way most toddlers, appropriately dubbed picky eaters, naturally behave. Sadly, by the time kids are school-age, they've lost this natural rhythm. Your job as your child's lean coach is to help him to relearn it.

Graze on Good Food

Let your child graze on foods that are high in fiber, yet have a low glycemic index. (The glycemic index measures how fast the food is absorbed in the bloodstream to trigger insulin release.) Grazing on junk foods, or foods that enter the bloodstream quickly, can keep insulin levels high and actually cause the child to get fat instead of lean.

MONITOR SNACKS

Since grazing is good for kids and children should get a lot of their calories from between-meal snacks, your job is to make sure their snacks are *nutrient dense* rather than *calorie dense*. Besides being tasty and nutritious, a lean snack should be satisfying—but not filling. It should satisfy a child's hungry tummy without creating the too-full feeling of a big meal.

That means lean snacks should be *fiber-filled* (contain at least three grams per serving), supply predominantly nutritious, *complex* carbs for energy, contain some protein and a bit of healthy fats, and preferably have a high water content. An average midmorning and midafternoon snack could be between 100 and 200 calories for a school-age child.

Not every food can accomplish all these goals. However, any food from the list below can be considered a good lean snack.

- Yogurt
- Carrot and celery slices (keep them cleaned and cut in your fridge) with hummus
- Cut-up apples, pears, bananas, and other fresh fruits
- Hard-boiled egg (keep a few in your fridge)
- Peanut butter on whole-wheat crackers
- Cheese slices on whole-wheat crackers
- Cherry tomatoes
- Air-popped popcorn
- Garbanzo beans (eat them like peanuts)
- Nuts, one palmful
- Edamane (Japanese soybeans)

An Open-Door Policy

Some children are actually challenged to eat more when you restrict their access to food. Others are emotionally scared by this kind of policy, and eat defensively. You're better off keeping an open-door policy to food. Just make sure your kitchen is filled only with nutritious foods. With lean eating, you seldom have to worry about a child eating too much.

DON'T NAG!

If you pressure your children to eat lean, they are more likely to eat fat. Food pressures override a child's natural appetite control cues. Avoid food wars. Even a time-honored enticement such as "You must eat your broccoli before you get dessert" runs the risk of making your child grow up to hate broccoli. Using too much pressure may also trigger eating disorders, overeating, or food aversions rather than food enjoyment.

Latch-key Leanness

When I was young—and fat—I was a latch-key kid. Since there is no one to supervise children's eating, activities, and screen time, home-alone children are at increased risk of getting overfat and underfit. To prevent this from happening, make junk food less available to your child. Purge the pantry and refrigerator of those temptation foods that unsupervised children are likely to overeat. Out of sight is out of mind, and therefore out of tummy. Leave healthy snacks readily available for your hungry after-schooler. Arrange after-school sports or community programs that provide supervision, exercise, and skill development.

Rather than lecturing your kids to eat lean, model lean eating. Simply don't buy junk food. Don't serve it, don't eat it, and don't have it in your house. Make lean food readily available. Display bowls of fresh fruit and veggies that serve as reminders: "This is the way to eat in our house." Eat them yourself with obvious enjoyment.

Peel Appeal

Oranges and pink grapefruit are great snacks. Besides being nutritious, the fruit must be peeled, which occupies a child's hands—a perk for the child who eats when bored.

HOLIDAY EATING

Want to get your children to try new foods or give them a veggie boost? Make holidays a theme for special cuisine. For example:

"For Valentine's Day we're going to eat foods that are good for the heart: salmon, sardines, salads, avocados, olive oil, and nuts."

"For St. Patrick's Day, let's try some great greens: swiss chard, spinach, arugula, kale, collard greens, and purslane."

"For Easter, let's eat eggs. I'll make a veggie omelet."

Throughout the year there are many holidays that can jump-start a finicky eater. Celebrating Groundhog Day may even spark an interest in sweet potatoes.

When you first start the LEAN Kids Program, you will want to follow our guidelines in explaining why you are doing it. But you should explain it only once to your child. Don't make it the only thing you talk about day in and day out. Only explain it again if your child asks, and keep your answers as short and specific as your child's questions are. It's important that children understand lean eating, but you won't teach them by lecturing them about it. Living it, and enjoying the natural good feelings it will generate, will teach them everything they need to know.

Let's Eat!

Chapters 9 and 10 cover a tremendous amount of information regarding nutrition. We hope they have given you a good idea of both what to eat and how to eat it. Our main goal was to help you understand that the LEAN Kids Program is not a restricted eating plan, like so many adult weight-loss programs are. Rather, lean eating is a whole new way of living. It is achieved through making a hundred small choices a day that lead to new and healthier habits. Don't try to master it all at once. Consider what is most important to you and your child. Take it one better decision at a time. You'll get there, and you'll feel better every step of the way.

CHART YOUR CHILD'S PROGRESS

Monitoring Success

Kids love tangible rewards. Nothing motivates a child to mow the lawn on a hot summer day faster than a promise that a visit to the pool will follow. From the little gold stars they earn in kindergarten to the A's they work for in middle school, kids love immediate recognition for their accomplishments.

This is the very reason why dealing with health issues can be so hard for some kids. Since the goal of the LEAN Kids Program is to maintain weight, some kids might feel frustrated by the absence of a clear-cut barometer to measure their progress as successful. Yes, I strongly believe that kids will come to enjoy food more and feel better when they live lean, but that kind of reward might be a little too subtle to motivate a child when she is just starting out on the plan. And, yes, I strongly believe that before too long your child will be running faster, shooting better baskets, and enjoying physical activities with his friends more. But those kinds of benefits just don't feel like rewards to kids.

So one of the most important jobs you have as your lean kid's coach is to provide him with the tangible recognition and rewards he needs. Explore ways to make her understand that even though she may not be losing pounds or waist-inches, each day she is making great strides by changing key lifestyle habits and the way she moves, thinks, and eats. The key is to find a way to recognize each new lean choice they make, each step they take in the right direction, each new habit they acquire.

Children love charts. Most kids love to collect points, stars, and ribbons, and see their progress displayed on charts. Records of this kind address their questions, "Have I reached the goal yet? How am I doing now?" in very tangible, visual ways. In this chapter, we'll review several different strategies you can use to track your children's progress and offer them the immediate gratification that they, as children, need. At the same time, we think you'll find that these projects will help you to bring together all the advice we've offered in the LEAN Kids Program and build a plan for your family's new way of living.

As we've discussed, the LEAN Kids Program can be narrowed down to four powerful goals:

1. Live Lean: Make wise, healthy choices.
2. Play Lean: Move one's body for thirty to sixty minutes a day.
3. Think Lean: Speak positively to oneself and others.
4. Eat Lean: Make nutritious choices.

Your goal is to change your child's and family's choices in these four areas. Our experience is that, if you concentrate on doing this consciously for twelve weeks, you will find your life transformed. Twelve weeks of choices will become a whole new set of habits that you no longer have to work at consciously. You will have achieved a whole new way of living.

To help you organize our lean advice into a program of choices that will build these habits, we recommend the following strategies. You might even want to use more than one. Let your child choose the one that works best.

Keep a Lean Journal

In our pediatric practice, we've found that children on the LEAN Kids Program who keep a journal feel more involved in the plan. They also seem to have a greater sense of ownership over their accomplishments.

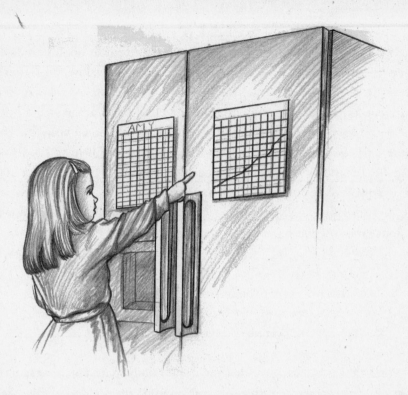

They make choices more deliberately and feel more involved in every aspect of the program. This is a strategy that's especially good for children who love to write and do so easily.

There are many different styles of journals. Here are some that our young lean participants find most effective.

A SIMPLE JOURNAL

Let your child choose a spiral-bound notebook and a pen. On each page, write in four headings: Lifestyle, Exercise, Attitude, and Nutrition. Leave a few lines blank under each of these headings, so that there's space to note specific lean choices made each day. The choices can be many or few. The journal can just serve as a place to keep a record of accomplishments made each day.

Lifestyle: _____

_____

Exercise: _____

_____

_____

Attitude: _____

_____

_____

Nutrition: _____

_____

THE DAILY INSTEAD-OF JOURNAL

If your child doesn't enjoy writing, you might prefer to give him a more structured journal. One that we've been very successful with is what we call the "Instead-of Journal." The first step to using this kind of record is to choose four goals. We think they should be fairly specific, and your child should probably try to choose one from each of the Lifestyle, Exercise, Attitude, and Nutrition chapters. These goals should be noted on the first page of a notebook. Then the child should assign a different day to each subsequent page, and simply note whether or not he accomplished his goal that day. Once he accomplishes a goal fourteen days in a row, he should replace it with a new goal.

Here's an example of what an Instead-of Chart might look like:

Instead of . . .	I will . . .	Today, I . . .
Eating potato chips while watching TV	Exercise while watching TV	I used my exercise band for 20 minutes
Playing video games after school	Join a softball team	During practice today, I played shortstop and got 2 hits
Being sad a lot	Think happy thoughts	I looked forward to my softball game
Skipping breakfast	Eat a healthy breakfast	I had yogurt, fruit, and whole-grain cereal

THE HIGH/LOW JOURNAL

Sean Foy, the fitness instructor to the kids on the LEAN Program in our pediatric practice, told me about a game his family plays each night. "After dinner our family plays a game called High/Low. No, it's not a card game! We all have an opportunity to share what was the best or high part of our day and what was the most disappointing or low part. It always makes for lively family discussion as well as some precious times of caring for and supporting one another."

We love this idea, and think it would be a great format for a lean journal for some children. It's especially good for children who like to be perfectionists, and need to be reminded that being lean doesn't mean you have to be perfect. It helps them understand that they can make mistakes and still make progress.

Unless your child really excels at writing, this is probably a journal that you should help him keep. In fact, I recommend that you let it grow out of a dialogue with you. Here's how it might work.

Start by sharing your own personal highs and lows on the LEAN Kids Program for the day. You might express what you are learning about yourself. For instance, you might say, "My goal was to run three miles today. I really didn't want to when I got up this morning, and I had a hard time making myself do it. But then when I was done, it turned out to be the most fun I've had running in a long time." You can explain to your child that you learned a lot from this experience. First, you experienced the low of not wanting to exercise. Then you experienced the high of having fun on your run. Most important, you learned that you shouldn't let an initial reluctance deter you from following through on your promise to keep with the LEAN Program—because when you do follow through, it feels great.

After sharing your own victories and challenges, ask your child, "How was your day?" See if you can get her to share a mistake and a victory in each of the four LEAN areas. It is very important to congratulate your child for even the smallest victory! Most children enjoy this family time to discuss their personal victories during the day or week. Coaches with "listening ears" are the most supportive and successful ones.

Here are some questions you might ask your child to help him understand what he can learn from his highs and lows:

- What did you learn from the situation?
- What can you think of that may help you next time a situation like this arises?
- What if one of your friends was going through this situation? What would you suggest for them?
- End by asking your child which of the solutions he thinks is best.

Finish this exercise by making note of your conversation in your child's High/Low Journal. We think you should devote one page to each of the four LEAN subjects—Lifestyle, Exercise, Attitude, and Nutrition.

On each page, reserve a section for noting the high, the low, and the solution you and your child discussed. Reserve one section for any other comments or insights your child might want to contribute.

THE "I CAN" LIST

After the first month on the LEAN Kids Program, ask your child to list all the things he "can do" now better than he could do before. You might want to update this list each month. The following is a list given to me by one of my patients, ten-year-old Max, after he started on the LEAN Kids Program:

- I CAN run faster
- I CAN ride up a mild hill
- I CAN ride up a really steep hill
- I CAN do a push-up
- I CAN jump higher

- I CAN pick better food choices
- I CAN think better
- I CAN eat less
- I CAN go longer without feeling tired
- I CAN get better grades

LIFESTYLE
"Highs": List your personal victories relating to your Lifestyle.
"Lows": List your personal challenges relating to your Lifestyle.
Solutions: List possible solutions.
Comments or Insights: List additional comments or insights.

EXERCISE

"Highs": List your personal victories relating to your Exercise.

"Lows": List your personal challenges relating to your Exercise.

Solutions: List possible solutions.

Comments or Insights: List additional comments or insights.

ATTITUDE

"Highs": List your personal victories relating to your Attitude.

"Lows": List your personal challenges relating to your Attitude.

Solutions: List possible solutions.

Comments or Insights: List additional comments or insights.

NUTRITION
"Highs": List your personal victories relating to your Nutrition.
"Lows": List your personal challenges relating to your Nutrition.
Solutions: List possible solutions.
Comments or Insights: List additional comments or insights.

Play LEAN Kids Olympics

Many children are inspired by competition. If your child loves to compete, you might want to chart his progress using an Olympics theme, giving your child daily, weekly, or monthly gold, silver, and bronze medals in recognition for accomplishing designated LEAN Kids goals. The more lean choices your child makes each day, week, and month, the more medals he can win.

PICK YOUR GOALS

To start with, you and your child should come up with a list of lean goals. We recommend you review the Lifestyle, Exercise, Attitude, and Nutrition chapters, and select the goals you both feel you need and want to concentrate on. Obviously, the choices you list will depend on what your habits have been until now and what you think you can and want to try to change first.

To start (in the first four-week period), you will be asking your child to make no more than four lean choices a day. We think you should come up with a list of four possible choices in each of the lean categories to give him ample opportunity to meet this goal. As time goes on, you can add more choices in each category. As you'll see below, it gets harder to earn medals as time goes on—so you'll want to give your child more choices and more opportunities to score points. In order to add to your choice list, we recommend that you sit down with your child after each four-week session and review this book for new goals you want to focus on.

WEEKS 1 TO 4 GOAL CHART (UP TO 4 PER DAY)

Lifestyle	Exercise	Attitude	Nutrition
1. Met moving-equals-screen-time goal	1. Walked to school	1. Named one good thing about myself	1. Tried one new lean food
2. Read labels with Mom at grocery	2. Attended team practice	2. Practiced one mini-meditation	2. Had a good breakfast
3. Helped Mom with shopping or list	3. Did 3 strength-building exercises	3. Did a mental turnaround	3. Practiced chewing 10 times each bite
4. Worked on school petition for better beverages	4. Did 3 stretches	4. Told a joke at dinner	4. Drank only water

See page 229 for an example of a goal chart you might use for the first four weeks of your Olympic games.

DEFINE YOUR MEDALS

Now that you and your child know the choices you'll be concentrating on, let's review the reward scale used in these Olympic games:

	GOLD MEDAL	SILVER MEDAL	BRONZE MEDAL
Weeks 1–4:	4 Lean Kids choices per day	2–3 Lean Kids choice per day	1 Lean Kids choice per day
Weeks 5–8:	8 Lean Kids choices per day	5–7 Lean Kids choices per day	1–4 Lean Kids choices per day
Weeks 9–12:	12 or more Lean Kid choices per day	7–9 Lean Kids choices per day	1–6 Lean Kids choices per day

DEFINE THE PRIZES

As you see, the whole idea of the LEAN Olympics is to build a stratified system of rewards. So the next (and to your child probably the most important) part of your planning is to decide on what the prize will be for winning each kind of medal.

Obviously, we recommend that the prize not be junk food! Rather, we think that you and your child should identify a favorite activity you can do together as a reward. What is a special treat to your child? Miniature golf, a movie, a visit to the beach or amusement park, a hike or bike ride? It would be nice if the treat were a lean activity, but your emphasis should be on rewarding your child and not on scoring more lean points. Maybe if your child manages to win a gold medal after the whole twelve weeks are completed, you could even let her choose the destination for a family vacation.

LET THE GAMES BEGIN!

Now you're ready to play! The trick is to keep an accurate record of what your child achieves each day, so that you can accurately track his score and reward his accomplishments. You'll find that many children love competing in this way, even when it's against themselves.

Here's a sample of what a first week of your score chart might look like:

	Monday	Tuesday	Wednesday	Thursday	Friday	Saturday	Sunday
Lifestyle							
1. Met moving-equals-screen-time goal	x		x		x		x
2. Read labels with Mom at grocery			x				
3. Helped Mom with shopping or list							
4. Worked on school petition for better beverages	x				x		
Exercise							
1. Walked to school	x				x		
2. Attended team practice				x			x
3. Did 3 strength-building exercises		x			x	x	
4. Did 3 stretches			x		x		

	Monday	Tuesday	Wednesday	Thursday	Friday	Saturday	Sunday
Attitude							
1. Named one good thing about myself		x					
2. Practiced one mini-meditation							
3. Did a mental turnaround				x			
4. Told a joke at dinner	x				x		
Nutrition							
1. Tried one new lean food					x		
2. Had a good breakfast	x				x		x
3. Practiced chewing 10 times each bite		x				x	
4. Drank only water			x			x	

Below is a blank form you can copy to use with your child. This chart is built to hold choices for all twelve weeks. We advise that you list four choices in each category for the first four weeks; eight choices in each category for the next four weeks; and twelve choices in each category for the final four weeks. You do not need to add all new choices each week; you can just add to existing ones if you prefer. That should be something you and your child decide together.

	Monday	Tuesday	Wednesday	Thursday	Friday	Saturday	Sunday
Lifestyle							
1							
2							
3							
4							
5							
6							
7							
8							
9							
10							
11							
12							
Exercise							
1							
2							
3							
4							
5							
6							
7							
8							
9							
10							
11							
12							

	Monday	Tuesday	Wednesday	Thursday	Friday	Saturday	Sunday
Attitude							
1							
2							
3							
4							
5							
6							
7							
8							
9							
10							
11							
12							
Nutrition							
1							
2							
3							
4							
5							
6							
7							
8							
9							
10							
11							
12							

PART THREE

PREVENTION AS PART OF THE CURE

THE LEAN PROGRAM IS GOOD MEDICINE

Planting a "Doctor" Within

As we have seen in the preceding chapters of this book, the LEAN Kids Program helps kids escape the three big risks in middle childhood: being overweight, underfitness, and unhappiness. If you follow the advice and guidelines described in the prior chapter for twelve weeks, you will certainly find you and your children better armed against all three of these risks. After the first twelve weeks, living lean will become easier (more of a habit), and you will find yourselves getting stronger, fitter, and happier every day.

Yet that's not all the LEAN Kids Program will do for you. Without any additional effort on your part, you will find that the LEAN Kids Program also carries huge benefits for your children in terms of protecting them against disease. In this last chapter, we'll look at how the LEAN Kids Program is the best preventive medicine you can find.

Health Costs of Obesity

If we asked you to choose the most common cause of death in Americans today, which would you pick? Heart disease? Stroke? Cancer? Diabetes? Obesity? The answer may surprise you; it's obesity. Why? Because obesity increases the risk of all these other fatal conditions. In fact, the medical acronym for obesity-related illnesses is **CHAOS**, because overfatness causes Coronary disease, Hypertension, Adult-onset diabetes, Obesity, and Stroke.

When it comes to overeating, gain doesn't come without pain. Obesity burdens nearly every system in the body and can lead to both specific diseases and general health problems.

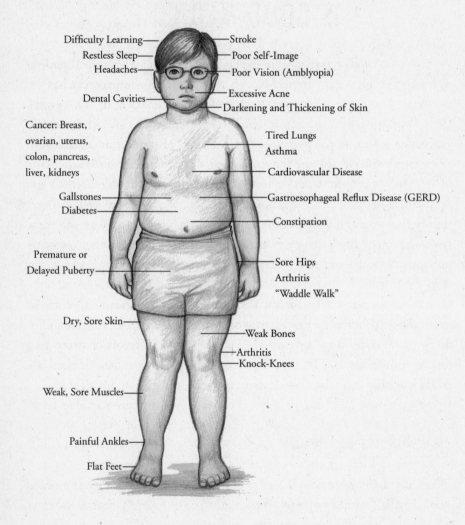

DISEASES OF OBESITY

Let's look first at some of the specific diseases that can directly result from obesity.

Early diabetes. Not only is the incidence of diabetes on the rise, it is occurring at younger and younger ages. Excess fat lessens the efficiency of insulin. Insulin escorts sugar from the bloodstream into the cells for energy, helping every cell in the body work efficiently.

By some biochemical quirk, obesity prevents the cells from listening to insulin. That means insulin has to shout louder (the pancreas has to produce more insulin) in order for the cells to let the sugar in. This eventually leads to type II diabetes, which doctors used to call "adult-onset" diabetes because they seldom saw it in children. Nowadays, it occurs even in preteens. As the child with type II, or insulin-resistant diabetes, grows older, the pancreas pours out more and more insulin and eventually wears out, leading to type I (or insulin-dependent) diabetes. What follows are the disease consequences of diabetes: the gradual wearing away of every system of the body, from blindness to failing kidneys. The overfat-underinsulin connection is dubbed *diabesity*.

Unhealthy little hearts. Excess body fat leads to excess blood fats. Obesity results in a triple whammy for little hearts: an increase in the LDL (bad cholesterol), an increase in total triglycerides (blood fat) levels, and a decrease in HDL (good cholesterol). While we think of coronary artery disease as an adult problem, fatty deposits have been found in children as young as eight years of age. The Bogalusa Heart Study, a landmark study of 14,000 children ages five to seventeen years, revealed an alarming fact: Compared with children of average weight, 58 percent of overweight kids already had risk factors for heart disease, such as high blood pressure and high cholesterol. Because of insufficient oxygen in the blood and the extra body fat it has to feed, the heart works harder by pumping more blood, eventually leading to high blood pressure and heart failure as the heart wears out. The obese child grows up with a constant case of "heart overload." While heart disease strikes in adulthood, it begins in childhood.

Tired little lungs. Imagine having to move an extra ten pounds of chest and abdominal fat every time you breathe. It's no wonder obese kids tire easily in sports. With the *obesity hypoventilation syndrome*, over-fat kids do not breathe deeply enough to inhale sufficient oxygen to meet their energy demands. Obese children are more prone to asthma. Due to their depressed immunity, when they do get a respiratory infection, it tends to be more severe.

Sore skin. Obese children tend to have dry, flaky, bumpy skin. They often get bacterial and fungal infections in the folds of skin that chafe together, especially in the neck, buttocks, and groin.

Gallstones. According to a study in *Pediatrics* in 2002, obesity-related gallbladder disease in children has tripled since 1980.

Weak little eyes. Ever wonder why so many obese kids wear glasses? The same nutritional deficiencies and excesses that affect all the other systems also affect their eyesight. With *nutritional amblyopia,* kids who eat excess junk foods are prone to vision problems.

Hurting little tummies. Obese children are prone to indigestion from GERD (gastroesophageal reflux disease, or what adults call "heartburn"). Presumably, reflux results from excess abdominal fat putting pressure on the stomach.

Sore little bones. Because of the extra weight that growing joints need to bear, obese children are prone to orthopedic problems of the hips, legs, and feet. Obese kids are prone to a condition called *slipped femoral epiphysis,* in which the leg bone slips out of the hip joint. The excess weight on growth plates (the softer and sensitive areas at the end of the leg bones) causes the bones to grow crooked, which makes obese children more prone to bowed legs and knock-knees. The combination of the excess weight supported by the legs and feet and the abnormal leg-bone development causes many obese children to have flat and sore feet. These sick bones limit the child's ability (and eventually his desire) to run, hop, and jump. Obese kids may "waddle walk." Overfat children are also prone to back pain. As a child grows into adulthood, this constant increased workload on joints makes her prone to arthritis and increases the chances of needing "spare parts," such as knee and hip joint replacements. Big bodies need big bones to support them. Even when overfat kids lean out, they often remain overboned. It may take years of eating right to lose that wide-body appearance.

HEALTH CONSEQUENCES OF OBESITY

In addition to the diseases that can result from obesity, your child's over-all health is worsened in a variety of ways if she is overfat.

Poor immune system. As we've discussed throughout this book, an overfat and underfit child is more likely to become a sick child who grows up to be a sick adult. That's because obesity depresses immunity. Specifically, it reduces the ability of white blood cells to fight infection. One study showed that fat children get twice as many infections as lean children. Children with depressed immunity get sick more often, and miss more school and more games.

Poor growth. Do you remember our four concerns from chapter 1? Children today are too fat, too sick, too sad, and too sedentary. Children must be well in order to grow. When children get sick, their growth systems shut down. They divert their energy into healing rather than growing. It stands to reason that the well child conserves more energy for optimal growth.

Restless nights, tired days. Excess fat accumulates in *all* areas of the body, not just the extra folds you pinch on your waist. Fat accumulates in the neck and tissues around the breathing passages, partially obstructing the airways and making it harder to breathe, a situation that can result in a condition called *sleep apnea*. In sleep apnea, a sleeping person stops breathing for twenty seconds or more and then takes a loud catch-up breath. The lack of oxygen will wake the sleeper up, but when he falls asleep again the cycle will repeat. In other words, people with sleep apnea don't get very much rest.

A combination of restless sleep and insufficient oxygen supply to the body interferes with the child's optimal growth. It leads to a tired child and poor school performance the next day. In Charles Dickens' novel *The Pickwick Papers,* Joe (the fat boy) was always falling asleep and would even fall off the carriage during the day. The combination of obesity, sleep apnea, and falling asleep during the day has been medically dubbed the Pickwickian Syndrome.

Tired little brains. Since the brain uses more oxygen than any other organ does, it stands to reason that the same breathing problems that cause a tired body lead to a tired brain. In fact, obesity-related sleep apnea can cause learning and behavior problems, leading to the child being tagged as having attention deficit disorder (ADD) or learning disabilities.

Puberty problems. Obese girls tend to begin puberty at a younger age. Their periods tend to occur earlier, yet be more irregular. Because excess body fat interferes with normal sexual hormone balance, obese girls may develop masculine features, such as rougher skin and coarser hair. Obesity is part of *Polycystic Ovarian Syndrome* (PCOS), a condition that can lead to infertility and diabetes. Obese males, however, tend to have delayed puberty. Possibly due to increased female hormones, obese boys often develop large, fatty breasts. Equally embarrassing for the obese male teen are the large pelvic fat folds that encircle the penis and make it appear small, or "hung-in" in teen talk.

Be Lean While You're Young

I wish someone had taught me how to live lean when I was young, and fat. The younger your child learns to live lean, the easier it is to stay lean. Studies show that obese children are more likely to become obese adults. If a child grows up lugging around a lot of excess fat during most of his childhood, the body interprets this excess as normal, which is why fat kids tend to become fat adults. Because the body tries to hold on to this excess fat, the child grows up feeling, "I just can't seem to shed this extra weight no matter how hard I try." The child who grows up lean has the advantage of the body interpreting leanness as normal, so the child's body is internally programmed to protect this leanness. The lean body interprets weight gain as abnormal. A lean child has a head start on growing up to be a lean adult. It's best to make lifestyle and eating changes while a child is still growing (and therefore is a natural calorie burner). Once the child stops growing, it's more difficult to stay lean.

Exercise As Preventive Medicine

Not only is a lean body good preventive medicine against disease, a lean *moving* body gives a child an extra dose. Let's look at all the healthful things regular exercise can do for you and your child.

HEALTH BENEFITS OF EXERCISE

Exercise builds a healthy heart. When your child moves his body regularly, his heart muscle becomes stronger and more efficient. The heart is like any other muscle: The more we use it, the stronger and more efficient it becomes. When we exercise regularly, our heart pumps at a lower *rate* and achieves a higher *stroke volume,* meaning that it moves more blood with each beat.

Because the heart of a regular exerciser is able to pump more blood with less effort, it's likely to last longer. Study after study confirms that regular physical activity helps clear the body of unhealthy fats that clog arteries and contribute to heart disease. Experts have found that nonexercisers have twice the risk of developing heart disease as individuals who exercise regularly.

Exercise builds strong bones. The growing years are the optimal time for the bone-strengthening effects of exercise. Since 90 percent of total bone mineral content is accumulated by the end of adolescence, optimizing bone mass and structure during childhood lessens the risk of broken bones in adulthood. Also, strong muscles help support our bones, giving us a stronger skeletal structure.

Exercise prevents injuries. Regular stretching exercises help children improve body posture and body symmetry, as well as minimize their muscular soreness after an activity or sport. Lengthening movements or stretching also prevents potential accidents and injuries by strengthening growing tendons and ligaments.

Exercise strengthens self-esteem. Kids who exercise regularly feel better about themselves than do kids who are couch potatoes. Researchers are finding that the more kids move their bodies, the more they experience higher self-esteem and general well-being.

Exercise fights depression. While we tend to think of anxiety and depression as adult mental problems, not surprisingly these diseases are occurring more frequently and at younger ages in children. Both aerobic exercise (brisk walking and running, for example) and strength training reduce depression. Fifteen to thirty minutes of exercise every other day can help depressed people enjoy frequent positive mood swings within two or three weeks.

Exercise strengthens social skills and enhances life skills. Students who participate in interscholastic sports are less likely to smoke or use drugs, and are more likely to stay in school and have good conduct and high academic achievement. Research also indicates that a lack of recreational activity may contribute to making kids more susceptible to negative influences such as drugs, gangs, or violence. Active sports and physical activity programs also have been shown to introduce kids to much-needed life skills, such as effective communication, leadership, teamwork, sportsmanship, conflict resolution, and goal setting. In a recent survey, many corporate executives said that they believed they owed much of their success to the skills they learned in team sports.

Exercise moves little bowels. Kids often get constipated, usually because they are too lazy or too busy to listen to their bowel signals. Moving the body moves the bowels, by speeding the transit time of intestinal contents.

Exercise builds smarter students. Regular physical activity can improve memory, enhance concentration, heighten imagination, and assist in creative thinking. Most likely this "smart effect" of exercise is primarily due to the enhancement of blood flow and oxygen to the brain.

Exercise helps children grow. Growth hormone, which is essential for building muscle, cartilage, and bone throughout the body, has been shown to increase a few minutes after exercise begins and to rise sharply when the intensity of the activity increases.

Exercise strengthens the immune system. Exercise perks up the immune system. Vigorous exercise stimulates the body to produce more infection-fighting white blood cells.

Exercise burns fat. Let's take a trip into your fat cells and marvel at how moving makes your body lean. The enzyme lipoprotein lipase (LPL) escorts fat from the bloodstream into fat cells for storage and into muscle cells for energy. Exercise stimulates a double biochemical benefit: It increases LPL activity (fat burning) in muscle tissue, yet *decreases* LPL activity (fat storing) in fat tissue. Inactivity, on the contrary, causes the reverse to occur: The body goes into fat-storing mode.

The Danger of Dieting Without Exercise

Fat loss and muscle gain must go together to achieve leanness. Dieting alone won't work! If you lose fat by dieting without simultaneously gaining muscle by exercising, you might end up actually gaining weight. As you lose fat by dieting alone, you can also lose some of the muscle that the body used to support the extra fat. As a result, the body's resting metabolic rate (RMR) diminishes, so you burn fewer calories as your dieting body clicks into anti-starvation, fat-storage mode. Yet, if you increase muscle at the same rate you lose fat, you keep the RMR revved up and can even increase it to continue burning rather than storing calories.

HOW MUSCLE IMPROVES HEALTH

While exercise in general improves health, building muscle in particular has a number of specific health benefits. Let's look at these one at a time.

More exercise equals stronger muscles. Our children's muscles are what help them sit, stand, breathe, walk, play, and live. All of the daily activities we frequently take for granted, such as combing hair, holding a pencil, running on a playground, kicking a ball, and raising an arm to ask a question, are possible because of muscle. Yet even with young children, *inactivity leads to muscle loss.* If you want your children to stay strong their entire lives and enjoy all the benefits good muscle tone gives them, you have to get them up and get them moving!

Burn Fat While You Sleep

The more you exercise, the higher your resting metabolic rate and the more fat the body burns, even in a resting state. Imagine burning more fat while you sleep! Your resting metabolic state can remain elevated for two to fifteen hours after a bout of exercise, creating a fat-burning body that continues to work long after the activity has stopped. What a lean perk!

More muscle equals less fat. How our body burns calories is primarily related to how much muscle we have. For every pound of muscle on the body, an individual expends (through fat burning) roughly 50 calories a day. So, if a child (or an adult) were to add two pounds of muscle to his body, he would increase his ability to burn energy by 100 calories a day. (That's ten pounds of excess fat burned in a year.)

Here's how it works: Sugar, the prime source of energy for a growing child, is stored in two fuel tanks in the body—the liver and the muscles. Sugar from the bloodstream is deposited in these tanks in the form of *glycogen,* the body's form of reserve fuel. Glycogen is composed of piles of sugar molecules linked together and released from this storage bank when needed.

The body has another large reserve tank: body fat. When a child eats excess sugar, it is first deposited in the liver as glycogen, and when this tank is full, the sugar is deposited in muscle glycogen. If the child eats more sugar than the muscle tank will hold, this excess is deposited in the reserve tank as body fat.

How do you keep the excess sugar out of the fat tank? Of course, the first answer would be to eat less of it. Yet it's also true that you can increase the capacity of the muscle storage tank so less sugar spills over into the fat tank. That's why the more muscle you have, the less likely your body is to store fat.

> ### LEAN KIDS SAY
>
> "The stronger I get, the more I can eat without getting fat."
> —JASON, AGE TEN

Muscle keeps you young. The physiological effects of inactivity are similar to those of *premature aging*, with a decrease in metabolism, happy hormones, and muscle strength and an increase in body fat, blood pressure and lipids, and aging. In fact, we doctors know that kids who sit too much grow old too fast. We also know that kids who are active and lean are healthier and experience optimal growth.

Junk Food Makes Junk Muscles

Teach your child that "you are what you eat." Two lean lessons made an impact on our children. In the supermarket, we showed them the difference between wild Alaskan salmon, which had a dark, rich color and a firm texture, and farm-raised salmon, which had a pale color (unless the fish was dyed) and a flaccid texture. I added, "See what happens to the muscles in fish when they are fed junk food and don't move around as much. They get flabby and weak. Notice how healthy and strong the muscle looks in the fish that eat healthy and exercise a lot."

To make this lean lesson stick, we then bought a piece of sirloin steak and cooked it along with some wild game meat a hunter had given us. The kids were amazed at the difference between the dense, healthy-looking muscle of the game that ate a "lean food diet" and the weaker-looking, fat-marbled muscle of the beef steer that was fed a junk-food diet. They got the point that lean food builds stronger muscles.

More muscle equals less diabetes. Muscles help prevent sugar spikes. If you haven't guessed it already, muscle is the body's way of handling our sugar cravings. As we have described above, when muscles soak up excess blood sugar, they also steady our blood-sugar levels. Because muscles soak up sugar better than fat tissue does, blood sugar tends to be steadier in a muscular person than in an obese person. Theoretically, fewer sugar spikes could decrease the risk of diabetes. Muscle helps the body to use insulin and glucose more efficiently. This could explain why muscular people tend to have a lower incidence of insulin-resistant diabetes.

Food As Preventive Medicine

Whole foods are whole medicine. One of the most important lean lessons we hope you have learned from this book is that factory foods are fake foods.

One of the most important things your child can learn from living the LEAN Kids Program is the idea that food is more than something to eat; it's actually preventive medicine. Everything we put into our body affects our overall health, and the younger your child is when she learns this fact, the healthier she'll grow. Let's look at how lean nutrition can boost your child's immunity to infection.

THE BATTLE WITHIN

To help your child make the connection between leanness and wellness, here's a story you can share on how the LEAN Kids Program can help his bodies fight nasty germs.

We live in a world full of nasty bugs that can make us sick. There are billions of bugs out there. Most of these bugs are so tiny you can't even see them. Tiny bugs are called germs. They come from people who are sick. They hang out in the air, on unwashed food, on people's hands, on doorknobs, and in unclean water. These germs like to get inside your body and make you sick. And the truth is, they get inside you all the time. Why aren't you sick all the time? Because your body fights back.

To fight these billions of bugs, your body has an army of fighters that attack these germs before they have a chance to make you sick. Just like the army that defends our country, this army has to be trained to fight. You have to give your army the best fighting equipment and feed the army powerful foods so it can keep you well. Let's meet each of these groups of fighters in your army.

The infantry on the front lines. Germs get into your body in three ways: through your skin, through your lungs when you breathe, and through your tummy when you eat. The skin, lungs, and tummy are on the front line of our war against germs. We help them by giving them good shields to use as protection. To keep the germs off our skin, we wash our bodies every day and we wash our hands before eating and after going to the bathroom. To keep the bugs out of our tummies, we wash fruits and veggies before eating them, and we cook meat (which kills the germs). To keep the germs out of our lungs, we breathe clean air and keep an arm's-length distance from kids with colds. (And to help keep our friends from catching our germs when we're sick, we always cover our nose and mouth when we sneeze or cough.)

No matter how well your army defends your front lines, some germs are bound to get through into your bloodstream and be carried all through your body by the rivers of blood inside. You need to keep the soldiers in your bloodstream well prepared, because that's where the real battle against germs takes place.

Your army's uniform. Let's imagine we shrunk ourselves into a tiny boat and traveled through the rivers of your bloodstream and watched your army in action. First, you would see many tiny soldiers called *white blood cells* that travel in packs, like schools of fish. Each white cell looks like a miniature Pac-Man that can gobble up germs. (In fact, the medical name for these Pac-Men is "macrophages"—meaning "big eaters.")

Sometimes there are so many germs that these Pac-Men can't gobble them up fast enough, so they call for reinforcements, or backup troops. These are special forces like Navy Seals. In fact, doctors call them "killer white cells."

Military housing. As we travel through your body in our little boat, we notice that all over your body there are many houses about the size of a pea. We'll call them the troop barracks. You can feel them like tiny bumps (doctors call them lymph nodes) in the back of your neck, under your arms, and in your groin. Sometimes when you get an infection, like a sore throat, you can feel these lumps get big and hard. When this happens, your body is mobilizing the troops to get ready for the battle against the germs in your body.

Command center. The generals in the army are able to talk with the troops using something that works sort of like the walkie-talkies you use to communicate with your friends in the neighborhood. When a germ enters your body, for instance through a scratch in your skin, the injured troops in the skin send a message to the command center in the nearest barracks. Special troops are dispatched in a search-and-destroy mission to kill the germs at the cut before they can sneak into the blood and really make you sick. These troops engage in a sort of chemical warfare (called dilating your blood vessels) to make the rivers of your blood larger so that troops can enter the battle. This is why your skin often gets red and swollen near the cut.

As we travel around in our little boat, we'll also see more chemical warfare. Special ground troops spray germ-fighting chemicals over the places where germs are most likely to enter: the lining of your breathing passages and the lining of your tummy. This stuff is like protective paint that coats the lining of your lungs and gut and keeps out the germs. The name of this paint is "immunoglobulins."

Know your allies. You should know that some good germs naturally live in your tummy. Doctors call them good bacteria. In return for a warm and safe place to live, these good bacteria coat the lining of your tummy and help your soldiers fight disease-causing germs.

The army remembers. The memory center of your army is very smart. Every time a new germ enters your body, the army keeps a record of how it fought and won the battle. So the next time a similar germ tries to invade your body, this army is already on alert. The weapons are ready. These special weapons are called antibodies.

Supply your troops. Feed your army well. Just as real soldiers need the best weapons to win a battle, the soldiers in your immune army need the strongest kind of fuel to fight. The foods we recommend on the LEAN Kids Program will give your soldiers the strongest weapons available. Junk foods will give your soldiers the kind of broken weapons that can blow up in their faces and do more harm than good.

That's why the LEAN Kids Program helps keep you from getting sick as a child and as an adult. The foods you eat to be lean are the same foods that arm your body to fight disease.

Pure Parents, Pure Kids

Over my three decades in pediatric practice, I have noticed a striking correlation between how children are fed and how they grow and behave. Early on in my practice I noticed a group of moms and dads who at that time would have been called "health-food nuts." I dubbed them "pure parents"—parents who would not let harmful foods and impressions pollute the growing bodies and minds of their children. Over the years I would notice that the "pure children" of "pure parents" were not sick as much as those in a "junk food" family. I would see them less during the usual cough and cold seasons. When they entered school they would get tagged with fewer labels such as ADD or learning disabilities. If one of these children did have one of these problems, he seemed to have a milder case and would cope better. The pure kids have the gift of the Wisdom of the Body, thanks to their pure parents.

THE BEST WEAPONS AVAILABLE

While all the foods recommended on the LEAN Kids Program help your child fight disease, certain foods are more helpful than others. In military terms, we would say that certain foods—health foods (or "grow foods," as discussed in chapter 9)—are better-armed soldiers for fighting germs than others.

That's because health foods contain natural biochemical antibiotics

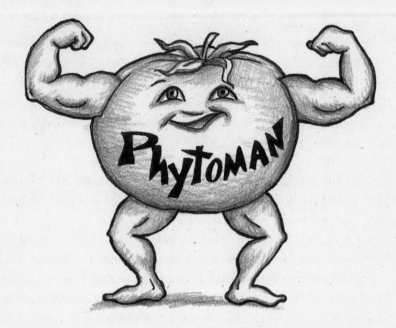

known as *phytonutrients*—we call them "phytos" for short. Phytos are what give fruits and vegetables their colors of blue, orange, red, yellow, and green. The darker the color, the better the phytos. That's why blueberries, tomatoes, pink (instead of white) grapefruit, sweet (instead of white) potatoes, and watermelon are all healthy phytos. Dark greens, such as spinach, have a lot more phytos in them than iceberg (or "see-through") lettuce.

Phytochemicals are also called *antioxidants.* Explain to your child that when his armies go to battle against germs, they make a big mess.

Watch Phytos Fight for You

Play show-and-tell. Cut an apple in half. Sprinkle lemon juice on the surface of one half. Examine the two apple slices in two hours. Notice how the lemon juice, which is full of phytos, protects the apple from turning brown (oxidation). That's how phytos protect your body from getting sick.

They produce lots of waste products (called "free radicals"), which can leave his equipment rusty—a biochemical reaction called *oxidation*. Phytos act like military garbage collectors who roam throughout the body and round up the waste products called free radicals that can get in the army's way. Phytos work as mechanics, helping the body to repair itself from environmental ailments, such as ultraviolet light, smoke, and pollutants. Phytos act like a protective antirust paint to keep the army's equipment from rusting.

Besides the phytos in fruits and vegetables there are lots of other health-building nutrients in nutritious foods. Let's look at each of them, and how they work.

Zinc increases white blood cells. Zinc, a vital mineral, increases the number of infection-fighting white blood cells and helps them fight more aggressively. Zinc is like a recruitment office, enlisting new soldiers in your army. The best resources of zinc for children are wheat germ, tofu, seafood, meat, poultry, nuts, and beans.

Omega-3 fats boost immunity. These healthy fats aid immunity by increasing the ability of white blood cells to eat up bacteria. They are like powerful machine guns to help your soldiers kill as many germs as possible. Omega-3s also help the body heal and repair itself. The best source of omega-3 fats are cold-water fish, such as salmon and tuna. Flaxseed and other lean oils are also good sources.

Vitamin C protects the immune system. While all vitamins are necessary for a protective immune system, vitamin C is particularly beneficial. It's kind of like the best gun you can give your soldiers. Best food sources of vitamin C are citrus fruits, peppers, guavas, kiwi fruit, and kale.

Vitamin E helps kill germs. Along with vitamin C, vitamin E helps white cells and assists these cells in producing antibodies that kill germs. Best food sources are sunflower seeds, sunflower oil, wheat germ oil, nuts, peanut butter, canola oil, olive oil, salmon, wheat germ, tomato purée, avocados, and vitamin E–fortified cereals.

Probiotics support healthy germs. Unlike antibiotics that the pediatrician prescribes to fight germs (when your soldiers need extra help), probiotics are naturally occurring tiny bugs that live in your body and actually support the healthy germs. The most familiar probiotic is *Lactobacillus acidophilus,* the main bacteria culture in yogurt and certain cottage cheeses.

Health Foods

When your child understands that choosing what to eat is like shopping for weapons to arm his soldiers, he might understand why the choices he makes are so important. Show him this "shopping list" to keep his army well supplied.

- Apples
- Blueberries
- Broccoli
- Carrots
- Chili peppers
- Citrus fruits
- Cranberry juice
- Fish (especially salmon)
- Flaxseeds, ground
- Garlic
- Legumes: beans and lentils
- Melons
- Papaya
- Pink grapefruit
- Pumpkin
- Red grapes
- Salmon
- Shiitake mushrooms
- Soy products
- Squash
- Sweet potatoes
- Tomatoes
- Yogurt

Planting a "Doctor" Within Your Child

You might be surprised to hear two doctors declaring that one of the best benefits of their program is that it will help you avoid doctors. Yet remember that the word "doctor" comes from the Latin word meaning "teacher." The LEAN Kids Program can be used by your doctor to teach you how to stay well. The LEAN Kids Program goes a long way in making your children so healthy that they don't get sick in the first place, and

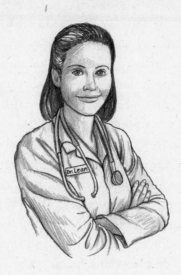

they're strong enough to fight off sickness when it does happen. And nothing makes us happier than the children we see only once a year for their annual checkup! In fact, we explain to kids that living and eating lean is like having a doctor inside you.

While living the LEAN Kids Program will go a long way in keeping you away from pediatricians like us, there are some other tips we can give you.

THE PROBLEM WITH PILLS

Ours is a culture growing increasingly dependent on medication to maintain our health, but (even as someone who makes his living prescribing pills!) I must say this is bad news. Of course, modern medicine has enabled many kids with debilitating diseases, such as diabetes, to lead functional lives. Yet pills are not without problems. Every medicine has uncomfortable side effects—some minor, some very unpleasant.

A worse problem with pills is that the body *habituates* to medicine. This means that the body gets so used to a medicine that the medicine often stops working, requiring a higher dose and bigger side effects.

Not only does the body habituate to medicine, but so does your mind. Many people immediately click into the pop-a-pill mind-set when a health problem occurs. This is not a healthy habit for your child to develop.

Use "medicine plus." A healthy alternative to pill-popping is a more responsible approach that I call "medicine plus." Teach your child, "Take your medicine, *plus* take care of your health." Home remedies are often as effective as prescription drugs in addressing some illnesses. Suppose your child has a cold or stuffy nose. Instead of (or in addition to) administering cold medicines, instruct your child to eat immune-boosting foods, "hose the nose" with saltwater nasal spray, and "steam clean" the sinuses using a facial steamer. These home remedies will help your child feel better without the cost of unpleasant side effects.

No matter what illness your child has and what medicines he needs, always advise him to do everything he can to help his body heal. Teach your children to *think themselves well*. One of the mysteries of medicine is how the mind can heal the body. With the "placebo effect," if a person takes a pill and convinces himself that the medicine will make him feel better, it sometimes will. For example, in some studies comparing children who took Ritalin pills with a group of children taking sugar pills or "placebos," 37 percent of the children taking the sugar pill showed improved behavior similar to the Ritalin group. When your children are sick, teach them to imagine themselves getting better!

BE SUPPLEMENT SAVVY

Many parents give their children daily multivitamin/multimineral (MV/MM) supplements as a nutritional insurance policy in case the children are deficient in any of these elements. Some parents feel that "it's simply easier to give my child a vitamin pill than to fight with him to eat his veggies!" Studies do suggest that a daily MV/MM supplement can improve the behavior, intelligence, learning, and general health of malnourished children.

Supplements are not substitutes. The important thing to keep in mind is that supplements are just that, supplements to overall good nutrition. Consider supplements in addition to, never instead of, a nutritious diet. It's better to get nutrients from foods rather than pills.

Just because the label claims the pill has a certain number of milligrams of a nutrient doesn't mean that same number will get *into the body*. Nor does the nutrient in the pill get into the body the same way that a nutrient would if it were packaged in a food. The nutrients in whole foods come packaged with substances that help your body utilize the nutrients more efficiently. Whole-food nutrients often have a *higher bioavailability* (how much of the nutrient gets into the bloodstream) than if that same nutrient were in a pill.

Also, keep in mind that the amount of each nutrient found in some vitamin supplements (see the ingredient list on the box) is often just the *minimal* level of the nutrient that the average child needs to keep her from suffering the disease of a particular deficiency. For instance, the recommended daily requirement for vitamin D is 400 I.U., an amount that has been determined to prevent rickets or weak bones. Yet, these numbers don't adequately reflect the amount of the nutrient that most children need for *optimal health*, which may be considerably higher than the number in the RDA (Recommended Daily Allowance) or DV (daily value) given on the box. This is why I prefer the term vitamin or mineral "insuffiency" rather than "deficiency" as a more accurate reflection of the current state of children's nutrition.

After surveying the medical literature, and guided by our own experience as pediatricians, we conclude that the most common nutritional deficiencies in children, and ones that may benefit from supplements, are:

- Omega-3 fats or long-chain polyunsaturated fatty acids (LCPUFAs)
- Iron
- Zinc
- Calcium
- Fiber
- Antioxidants (Phytos)

If you are going to give your child any supplement, we would advocate one that provides these nutrients. But the greatest gift you can give your child is to teach him that healthful living—making the right choices about what foods to eat—is the best possible medicine. (See www.LEAN KIDS.com/supplements for updated information.)

The LEAN Kids Program Prevents More Than Disease

The LEAN Kids Program is not only good prevention against disease, it's good preventive medicine against the harmful habits that lead to disease. Because this program helps children resume their Wisdom of the Body, it's likely that these children will shun unhealthful habits such as smoking, drugs, and other temptations that can harm their health. Some kids on the LEAN Kids Program have told me, "How can anyone put that stuff in their body?" referring to smoking. I've witnessed adults on the LEAN Program quit smoking because, for the first time in their lives, they now perceive this habit as completely foreign to their body.

The Gift of Health

In closing, we would like to reiterate that we have written this book in the hope of improving the quality of life for both you and your child. Science has shown us that leanness increases longevity. Sadly, we live in a culture that does not encourage leanness as the norm. It is a state of health that you have to consciously make an effort to achieve.

We hope that in the course of this book, we have given you the information you need to live a longer, stronger, and happier life. We hope we've shown you a way to share this knowledge with your children. We strongly believe that one of the most valuable legacies you can leave your children is the gift of health. We hope that, in this book, we have provided everything you need to live lean and bring this gift to your entire family.

LEAN KIDS PROGRAM REVIEW

The following list is a wrap-up of some important lean living and eating reminders. Check the ones you regularly do and try to improve on the ones you don't.

DO YOU?	HOW TO, PAGES:
☐ Limit sweetened beverages?	179–181
☐ Limit foods with hydrogenated oils?	185
☐ Encourage your child to exercise 30–60 minutes daily?	245
☐ Choose LEAN-living caregivers?	101
☐ Nurture happy thoughts?	160
☐ Encourage muscle-strengthening and lengthening exercises?	137 and 127
☐ Begin meals with high-fiber salads?	115
☐ Order kids' food from adult menus at restaurants?	116
☐ Lobby for lean foods at school?	119
☐ Enforce the "sitting equals moving" rule?	145
☐ Serve salmon at least twice a week?	172, 186
☐ Buy organic foods?	165
☐ Serve lean protein foods?	172
☐ Serve high-fiber foods?	176
☐ Serve dark greens instead of iceberg lettuce?	178
☐ Serve whole grain instead of processed cereal?	183
☐ Serve whole wheat instead of white bread?	115
☐ Serve brown or wild rice instead of white rice?	183
☐ Serve water instead of sweetened beverages?	191
☐ Serve a brainy breakfast?	201
☐ Try Dr. Bill's Schoolade smoothie?	206
☐ Offer smaller servings and refill as necessary?	208
☐ Remind children to chew their food longer?	209

DO YOU?	HOW TO, PAGES:
☐ Remind children to slow down and enjoy their food?	211
☐ Eat family meals together frequently?	212
☐ Not let your child munch while watching TV?	213
☐ Monitor snacks and make nutritious ones available?	216
☐ Teach your child smart supermarket shopping?	113
☐ Help your child chart progress in a lean journal?	221

INDEX